Perfect Skin

perfect
skin

Perfect Skin

A Natural Approach

AMANDA COCHRANE

PIATKUS

⌘ Visit the Piatkus Website! ⌘

Piatkus publishes a wide range of exciting fiction and non-fiction, including books on health, mind, body & spirit, sex, self-help, cookery, biography and the paranormal. If you want to:

- read descriptions of our popular titles
- buy our books over the internet
- take advantage of our special offers
- enter our monthly competition
- learn more about your favourite Piatkus authors

visit our website at:

www.piatkus.co.uk

First published in 2000 by
Judy Piatkus (Publishers) Limited
5 Windmill Street
London W1T 2JA
e-mail: info@piatkus.co.uk

The moral right of the author has been asserted

A catalogue record for this book is available from the British Library

ISBN 0 7499 2113 7

Design by Jerry Goldie Graphic Design
Edited by Anne Lawrance

This book has been printed on paper manufactured with respect for the environment using wood from managed sustainable resources

Data manipulation by Selwood Systems,
Midsomer Norton
Printed and bound in Great Britain by
Butler & Tanner Ltd, Frome, Somerset

CONTENTS

Acknowledgements

My thanks go to all those who have so generously shared their knowledge with me – to Danièle Ryman for introducing me to the world of aromatherapy all those years ago; Katherine Jackson who integrates Eastern wisdom into her natural skin treatments and makes the most wonderful home-made face masks; Eve Lom for her inspirational approach to skincare; and Kitty Campion for revealing the power of natural therapy.

I would particularly like to thank my agent Teresa Chris for her encouragement and commitment to this book; to Rachel Winning, my editor at Piatkus, for her genuine enthusiasm and guidance; and to everyone who volunteered to test my skin creams and were brave enough to give their honest opinion.

Finally, a big thank you to Jeremy, Hamish and Kitty for giving me the time and space to write this book. Without your understanding and patience it would never have been possible.

Introduction

Perfect skin is never out of fashion. Since time immemorial
women all over the world have dedicated themselves to the pursuit
of amazing-looking skin.

Most of us envisage perfect skin as being soft as satin and silky smooth, rather like rose petals in delicate shades and blushes of pink: it is fresh, vibrant and free from any blemishes. In reality skin rarely attains such perfection.

This is because skin is not simply a cosmetic covering. It is a complex living organ that is intricately connected to other bodily systems, and as such it mirrors your sense of wellbeing. Nowadays, ever-present stress, high levels of pollution and diets depleted of certain nutrients mean our skin rarely looks or feels as good as it could.

Ever since I began working as a beauty journalist I have been intrigued by the possibility of improving the quality and texture of skin from within as well as without. I noticed how my skin reflected how I felt, both emotionally and physically. If I was stressed out and run down my skin lost its vitality and behaved in unexpected ways.

Spots almost always appeared around the same time every month suggesting that hormones, rather than insufficient cleansing, were the problem. There were also times when my skin looked and felt fantastic – usually after a holiday in the country or by the sea. I wanted to know what I could do to keep my skin looking and feeling this good all the time.

Over the last 20 years I have experimented with a vast variety of different skincare preparations and explored all kinds of natural and complementary therapies. It became increasingly clear to me that the secret of perfect skin lay in achieving a sense of balance. This is not a new idea.

Thousands of years ago wise men living in India and the Far East proposed that perfection is a reflection of harmony. And, the only way to achieve this kind of equilibrium is to know yourself inside out.

We may share similar traits, but each one of us is unique and the same holds true for our skin. In other words what's good for one person will not necessarily suit another.

The time has come for a fresh approach to caring for skin that respects our individuality and works in a much more holistic way. That said, there are certain basic essentials that every skin needs to keep it healthy and looking good. They are:

Purity ~ Impurities and toxins prevent skin functioning smoothly, while airborne pollutants accelerate skin ageing.

Moisture ~ Essential for life and responsible for skin's softness.

Oxygen ~ Keeps the skin looking fresh and full of vitality.

Nutrients ~ These are used to create and nurture skin cells. Certain nutrients also offer protection from the age-accelerating effects of pollution and the sun's ultraviolet rays.

There are also things that upset the equilibrium, the most potent being stress which undermines skin's sense of wellbeing in a variety of different ways. The frantic pace of life, pressures at work and demands at home – to name just a few sources of stress – mean that our skin never quite reaches its potential for perfection. But there are ways to counteract the negative influence of stress.

Natural therapies like massage, hydrotherapy, herbal remedies, superfoods and plant essential oils have amazing powers for assuaging the ill-effects of stress and generally boosting natural vitality from deep within.

Qualities such as clarity, softness and radiance can also be cultivated with the right kind of skincare. My personal preference is for preparations made with pure, natural, organic ingredients. Why? Because they provide skin with the kind of nourishment it needs to look and feel its best. Herbs and essential oils, for example, contain active elements that help to balance certain skin activities such as how much oil the sebaceous glands produce and maintaining skin's natural protective barrier. Research in the field of cosmetology now reveals that some of the oldest natural beauty treatments have scientific credibility. Milk, for example, contains proteins that have an unbeatable ability to stimulate the synthesis of new collagen which helps to keep skin looking young.

I also worry that over-exposure to synthetic or man-made chemicals is harmful to health and detrimental to our skin. Twenty years ago skin sensitivity was relatively unknown. Now more than 50 per cent of women believe their skin is sensitive and over-reactive. Certain substances commonly used in skincare products such as preservatives, are known irritants likely to trigger allergic reactions and skin rashes. Synthetic fragrances and colourants are key culprits too.

One of the best ways to avoid these ingredients is to make your own organic, plant-based skin preparations. I have always enjoyed making simple things like masks made from yoghurt and fresh fruit, but was intimidated by the thought of making a cream. Then a few years ago I took the plunge. Some of my earliest efforts were thick and glutinous so I experimented endlessly, using different quantities of ingredients, and eventually produced some really lightweight creams and lotions that are a pleasure to use.

Throughout this book you will find recipes for all the preparations you will need to keep your skin in perfect condition. Making your own preparations also means you decide what goes into them. Just turn to Skincare Essentials (Chapter 12) to discover which herbs, flowers and essential oils are best for your skin right now. Making your own fresh skincare is economical too. Most natural ingredients are inexpensive. Essential oils will be the most pricey items on your shopping list, but remember you only use a few drops at a time and a small bottle contains enough to make countless jars of cream.

As your skin finds its own natural balance, problems such as excess oiliness, dryness and sensitivity should start to disappear, which means you no longer need all those corrective products on your bathroom shelf.

So go ahead, take the plunge – let nature unleash your skin's inner beauty.

balance

CHAPTER ONE

Blueprint
for
Perfection

~

There's an ancient belief that everything in nature has a blueprint for perfection. It's expressed in the unfurling petals of a rose, in the exquisite design of a butterfly's wings, in the crystalline patterns of snowflakes. Perfection, mused wise men of old, is the reflection both of inner balance and harmony with the natural world. To bring out skin's inherent beauty, we must know how to achieve that essential balance. But first we need to understand our skin. Self-knowledge is the key to fulfilling skin's potential for perfection.

Be enlightened.

The Nature of Skin

Your skin is amazing. Although it can be as soft and smooth as finely
woven silk or cashmere, skin is surprisingly tough and resilient.

Seeing skin as simply a yardstick for measuring beauty undermines the many important roles it plays. Skin is not just a cosmetic covering. It is an immaculately designed, living, breathing, hard-working tissue that acts as a highly perceptive go-between between us and the outer world.

HOW SKIN WORKS FOR YOU

Protective clothing

Your skin is a waterproof coat. Splash water on to your skin and the droplets will sit or slither off the surface. A healthy and well-balanced skin also retains the precious moisture that makes it soft and fresh-looking. But be aware that many substances, especially the oil-soluble variety, penetrate the skin's outer defences. Increasingly, drug companies are using skin as a medium for delivering hormones and other kinds of medication into the body. As skin may soak up harmful as well as helpful chemicals, it is essential to use the purest, most wholesome skincare preparations.

Keeping cool

The body works best when its internal temperature is kept at a constant 37°C (98.4°F). If the outside temperature soars, skin works overtime to keep us cool. The sweat glands produce more perspiration and as these beads of liquid evaporate into the air, the excess heat is lost and our temperature comes back down.

The subtle sense

Within the skin lies a network of complex sensory nerve endings which provide us with information about the outside world. Skin senses pleasure and pain through these nerves and relays them to the brain. Touch enriches our perception and adds another dimension to what we can see and smell. The desire to feel softness – the brush of cashmere against our skin, touching a rose petal – may spring from babyhood. It rekindles the sense of comfort and security that came from nestling against our mother's skin. Psychologists refer to the need to touch another's skin as 'skin hunger'. Science now supports the long-held notion that touch therapy or massage works wonders for the mind, body and soul.

Pathway to purity

Along with the lungs, liver, kidneys, lymphatic system and large intestine, the skin acts as an organ of elimination and works to rid the body of any unwanted substances. As well as salts, other substances may be carried away in perspiration.

If any of the other eliminatory channels are not working as efficiently as they could, the skin may find itself overwhelmed with more than its fair share of wastes. Spots are often a tell-tale sign that skin is trying to clear away its excess toxic load. Luckily there are many ways to help the skin to keep you clean.

In-built sunshield

Skin offers protection from some of the harmful effects of the sun's ultraviolet (UV) rays. Just how much protection it offers depends on your capacity to produce melanin, the dark pigment that gives us a tan. This is something determined by genetics. Fair skins are inherently more susceptible to the sort of sun damage that leads to wrinkles and age spots. But let's not forget that sunlight falling on the skin also triggers the synthesis of vitamin D, an essential nutrient needed for keeping the bones and joints healthy.

Reaping the benefits of sunlight without letting it damage and prematurely age our skin is a perfect example of getting the right balance (see page 133).

Chemistry of attraction

Everyone's skin has its own unique and subtle scent. The apocrine glands, which are concentrated under the arms, around the nipples and genital area, secrete tiny quantities of a milky substance containing substances known as pheromones. Although most of us are not aware of their aroma, these molecules do influence those around us. Female pheromones are thought to provoke sexual interest or arousal in men, especially around the time of ovulation and vice versa. Synthetic imitations have been added to perfumes designed to provoke desire, but why bother when you can make the real thing? Pheromones undoubtedly play a part in the complex chemistry of attraction, so it's not a good idea to smother them with synthetic perfumes. Better to cleanse away the bacteria that turn them sour and use the subtler scents of plants to enhance their allure.

— Tip —

Take good care of your skin and it will look after you too

Skin's Architecture

Skin has two distinct layers. The outer epidermis is the skin's protective covering. It is made up of layer upon wafer-thin layer of tiny cells.

The epidermal cells are born in what is known as the basal layer which lies at the bottom of the epidermal bed. They begin life as soft, plump cells laden with moisture. Then, like bubbles rising through water, they move up towards the skin's surface making a tough protein called keratin (the same stuff found in hair and nails) on the way.

By the end of their journey, these cells are dried-out, flaky shells of their former selves. Glued together with a waxy intercellular substance, they form the outermost stratum corneum. When the cells are tightly packed and lying flat, this layer forms an effective water- and germ-resilient barrier. Light bounces off evenly, giving skin a fresh and luminous appearance. Each day the oldest cells are sloughed away and new ones rise to take their place.

The rate at which new cells are formed and rise to the surface slows down with age. Teenage skin renews itself every two to three weeks but in our fifties it may take twice as long. But approximately every 28 days a new skin is born, giving us endless opportunities to attain perfection.

THE SPRING WITHIN

The epidermis rests on a part of the skin known as the dermis which acts as a cushion. In the dermis there are two kinds of fibre – tough, resilient collagen and supple, stretchy elastin – woven together to create a springy support system.

These fibres are made by specialised cells known as fibroblasts. As we age the collagen and elastin fibres stiffen and deteriorate and these changes are primarily responsible for causing wrinkles.

The dermis is home to the oil-secreting sebaceous glands which open on to the skin's surface through tiny pores. It also houses our sweat-secreting eccrine glands and the odour-emitting apocrine glands. The dermis is richly supplied with nerve receptors, making it highly sensitive to temperature changes and other kinds of sensory stimulation. It is fed by the thinnest blood capillaries which bring life-sustaining oxygen to the skin cells, then whisk away carbon dioxide and other cellular wastes.

VEIL OF PROTECTION

In a well-balanced skin, the oily substance secreted by the sebaceous glands and micro-beads of perspiration from the eccrine glands mingle to form a protective oil-in-water emulsion which acts as a natural moisturiser. Ideally skin responds to changes in humidity and temperature to create exactly the right oil and water combination needed to keep skin soft and smooth. This mantle has a slightly acidic pH value of around 5.5 which favours the presence of so-called commensal or 'friendly' bacteria that help to protect our skin from invasion by other pathogenic micro-organisms.

The best skincare regimes are those that don't overwhelm or destroy this protective mantle.

THE VOLUPTUOUS LAYER

Lying below the dermis is the subcutaneous fatty layer. As well as providing a useful layer of insulation, this fatty tissue gives skin its smooth and sensuous contours. Before reaching the dermis, nerves supplying hair follicles, sweat glands and skin receptors weave their way through the underlying fat cells. Here, too, lie the larger blood-carrying arteries and veins that branch into the tinier capillaries which feed the skin with oxygen and other nutrients.

This tissue is bathed in a clear lymph fluid which clears away cellular debris and wastes. Skin begins to look puffy if anything interferes with this inner cleansing.

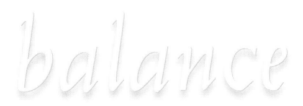

Knowing Your Skin

Each one of us is unique and this individuality is mirrored in our skin.

Some skin traits tend to run in families. You may have inherited your mother's fragile complexion which means your skin may be especially prone to fine lines. But a predisposition is just that. What you eat, how you respond to stress and how you care for your skin will ultimately determine how good it looks and feels. To bring out the best in your skin you need to recognise its inherent tendencies and learn its ways. The ultimate aim is to achieve a sense of balance.

BEAUTY THROUGH BALANCE

Thousands of years ago, wise men living in the Himalayan mountains came to believe that inner balance held the key to wellbeing in mind, body and spirit. It is the underlying principle of Eastern philosophies and healthcare systems including Ayurveda and Traditional Chinese Medicine. To be balanced is to feel energised yet relaxed; to be fired with enthusiasm yet inwardly at peace. Skin delights in this state of equilibrium. It looks radiant, glowing and younger than its years. But inner balance is constantly under threat from stress and tension, pollution, a nutrient-depleted diet and much more besides. Luckily there are

ways to restore and maintain a sense of balance, as you will discover in the following chapters.

EXPRESSIONS OF IMBALANCE

There is a tendency to classify skin as oily or dry, sensitive or spotty, but such problems are not set in stone. They suggest that something is out of kilter. The skin reflects our inner health and something is clearly amiss when it lacks vitality or breaks out in a rash. You can invest in the most expensive high-tech cream or treatment money can buy but unless you help your skin from the inside it will never perform miracles.

Oily or over-stressed? ~ Skin becomes oily when the sebaceous glands go into overdrive. These oil-producing glands are goaded into action by masculine hormones known as androgens which even women have in small amounts. All the body's hormones are kept in balance by the hypothalamus, an area of the brain that can be upset by stress. Excessive pressure at work, the strain of a bad relationship, exam nerves or even jet travel may lie at the heart of an oil crisis.

A poor diet, too many stimulants such as

coffee, and using harsh, oil-stripping cleansers can exacerbate the condition.

Daily relaxation helps to rebalance the hormones and an aggression dispersing exercise such as tae bo can provide a vent for those dynamising androgens. Foods rich in vitamins E, B2 and B6 can reduce oiliness, while skincare preparations incorporating herbs such as comfrey, sage and peppermint help to pacify and regulate those agitated sebaceous glands.

Dry or under-nourished? ~ Skin becomes dry when moisture evaporates too readily from the cells into the atmosphere. Dry skin is more common from the mid-thirties onwards because the sebaceous glands start producing less of the oil that goes to make up your natural moisturiser. Skin creams can replace this protective layer, but they only gloss over the problem.

To retain their precious moisture, skin cells must have strong, water-resistant membranes. These cell membranes are constructed from essential fatty acids, vital nutrients that help to moisturise skin from deep within.

Sensitive or overwhelmed? ~ Characterised by a tendency to break out in blotches and red rashes, skin flares up at the slightest provocation. Opting for hypo-allergenic skincare and cosmetic

preparations can reduce skin's exposure to irrtants. But what your skin really needs is strengthening from within. Sensitivity is a sign that your body is trying to cope with more toxins than it can handle. They may come from your diet, medication or environmental chemicals.

An holistic approach involves clearing away impurities and boosting your natural defence systems. Choose organically grown foods rich in antioxidant nutrients such as vitamin C, beta-carotene, vitamin E and zinc which help to boost your protection against pollutants from within. Black grapes, blueberries and cherries are rich in flavonoids, phytonutrients with antioxidant and anti-inflammatory properties. Soothe skin with simple organic preparations that harness the calming and fortifying properties of plants such as camomile, lavender and frankincense.

purify

CHAPTER TWO

Purity

~

The Essence of Crystal-clear Skin

P urity is the first step on the path to perfection. Clean skin has an aura of clarity that even the cleverest make-up cannot re-create. In a world where pollution is omnipresent, keeping your skin fresh and crystal-clear demands a cleansing regime that works both inside and out. Rituals of washing and polishing work in synergy with regular deep-cleansing treatments to keep the skin free from every kind of impurity. Your skin revels in being clean, so make a fresh start.

Be purified.

The Nature of Cleansing

A good cleansing ritual forms the basis of any skincare regime.
Whether your skin seems oily or dry, keeping it clean is an essential
step towards improving its quality and appearance.

Here's why. The natural oils that help seal moisture in the skin also attract tiny specks of dust and other particles in the air. The same is true of any moisturising or nourishing cream worn throughout the day and night. The more polluted the atmosphere, the dirtier the skin is likely to become. As well as airborne dirt, any salts and wastes left behind when micro-droplets of perspiration evaporate from the skin gather here too. Flaky skin cells that cling to the surface instead of being sloughed away add to accumulating dirt and wastes.

Left to linger on the skin, this debris dulls the complexion and clogs the pores, encouraging the formation of blackheads and spots. And as even featherweight make-up contains some oils and pigment particles, it will inevitably add to the skin's unwanted load.

THE ELEMENTS OF CLEANSING

Cleansers come in many forms – from soaps and foaming liquid washes to lotions and rich creams. But which one is best for your skin?

This depends on its ingredients. We are only now beginning to appreciate what French beauty experts have known all along. Skin has a natural empathy for pure plant preparations. Cleansers made from the purest vegetable oils and plant extracts are not only gentle and effective, but also free from synthetic chemicals which may disrupt the skin's natural functions.

THE BEAUTY OF BUBBLES

Nothing leaves your skin feeling quite as squeaky clean as soap and water washing. The light, frothy lather dissolves oils, dislodges dirt and loosens dead skin cells so the whole lot can be rinsed away.

So why has soap had such bad press? Concerns spring from soap's alkaline pH which can disturb the skin's acid mantle, leaving it susceptible to moisture loss and easy prey to harmful bacteria. But soaps vary enormously. There's a vast difference between commercial soaps made from animal fats and perfumed with synthetic scents which may indeed dehydrate the skin, and those made from good-quality, nourishing vegetable oils like olive and avocado with the fresh scent of pure essential oils.

Soaps containing 70 per cent olive oil are so lubricating that they cleanse without drying the skin. Any disturbance in pH value is quickly corrected by spraying the skin with a mildly acidic toner (just add a few drops of lemon juice or cider vinegar to your floral water, see page 22). Splashing the skin at least ten times with pure, preferably spring water removes soapy residues which may cause irritation. When taking a bath, spray your body all over with fresh water before patting dry with a towel.

If you don't like the feel of vegetable-oil soap, a clear glycerine-based variety may be a better option. Glycerine has humectant or water-attracting properties that keep the skin soft and moist.

Foaming gels and lotions can be made to match the skin's pH but some rely on strange-sounding chemicals to do so. Most skin washes contain varying amounts of an oil-dissolving ingredient called sodium lauryl sulphate which doubles as an industrial detergent (see page 195). The best preparations are primarily a mix of herbal infusions (see page 187), vegetable oils and plant extracts, with minimal amounts of this foaming agent.

– The perfect cleansing ritual –

Early morning – A simple one-step cleanse should sweep away the natural secretions and impurities that have accumulated during the night, plus any residues of a night-cream.

Choose a light plant-infused lotion such as home-made **Scented Milk** or **Skin Fresh Lotion** or a natural vegetable soap to suit your skin.

Late evening – At the end of the day, cleansing has to clear away natural skin wastes, any traces of moisturiser and residues of make-up.

A two-step approach works best to ensure your skin is scrupulously clean before bedtime. Use a cleansing milk or richer cleansing cream, both of which you can make yourself, to melt away oil-soluble residues and tailor to your skin's individual needs using a combination of herbal infusions and essential oils. To leave your skin feeling completely refreshed, follow this step with a gentle wash using a vegetable soap or sweep the skin with a gentle cleansing lotion.

Quick cleanse – For freshening up at any time in the day, spray your skin with a light floral refresher (choose one without alcohol) or make your own (see pages 22–3 for recipes).

CREAMY COMFORT

Cool creams and lotions that literally melt on the skin may feel like a luxurious option but they have impressive deep-cleansing powers.

This is because they have both an oil and water phase. Old, oily secretions become suspended in the oil phase while water-soluble wastes dissolve in the water phase. Everything can then be swept away with a warm, damp muslin cloth. This gently buffs away dead skin cells and leaves skin feeling wonderfully clean.

The best preparations are blends of pure vegetable oils and either pure spring water or a herbal infusion (see page 187) which can be chosen for its astringent (oil-removing), soothing, stimulating or antiseptic properties.

Creams and lotions contain the same basic ingredients of oil and water (or infusion) in differing proportions. These are blended together using emulsifiers such as beeswax and cocoa butter. They are unbelievably simple to make. The trick is getting a blend that creates the kind of consistency you prefer.

Many commercial cleansing creams and lotions are, on the other hand, made with mineral oil and other synthetics. Although this light, fine oil creates nice textures, it is derived from petroleum. Unlike vegetable oils which are rich in essential fatty acids, vitamin E and other phytonutrients, mineral oil has no nutritional value and may even leach away some of the skin's own fat-soluble nutrients. Petroleum derivatives also act as xeno-oestrogens (see page 116) which may be taken up by the skin.

Milk is nature's perfect oil-in-water emulsion. It contains lactic acid which gently dissolves away dead cells and maintains skin's natural pH, making it a mild but effective cleansing lotion.

For a simple morning cleansing milk, simply steep your favourite flower petals or a herb to suit your skin in a little milk (see **Scented Milk** recipes, page 21) and wipe over the skin. Use organic milk if possible.

– Tip –

Remove soaps, milks and creamy cleansers with a clean square of muslin dampened with warm water or a soft natural sponge.

– Harmonising essential plant oils and herbal infusions –

Use this chart for guidance when choosing or making a cleanser to suit your skin.

	ESSENTIAL OILS	INFUSIONS
Normal	rose, geranium	comfrey, lemon balm, rose petals, lime flowers, jasmine flowers
Oily	lavender, lemon, sandalwood	lavender, marigold, yarrow, sage, rosemary
Dry	geranium, camomile	elderflower, camomile, meadowsweet
Sensitive	sandalwood, frankincense	marshmallow, lady's mantle

HERBAL SOAPS

Making your own soap from scratch is tricky and time consuming. There are some wonderful pure soaps around that are hard to beat, but you might like to try grating down some pure, unscented vegetable soap and blending it with your own flower or herb infusion. To about 115g (4oz) soap gratings, add 1 cup of infusion and heat in a bowl over a saucepan of boiling water until it turns into a thick paste. At this stage you can add some honey for extra softness or oatmeal to make an exfoliating bar, and up to 8 drops of your favourite essential oil. If you are using a rose petal infusion, enhance the perfume with some rose otto. Spoon the mixture into a mould – seashells and star shapes are fun – and leave overnight to set. Turn out of the mould, wrap in greaseproof paper and store in the airing cupboard or another warm, dark place for a few days.

Making Your Own Cleansers

❧ Make small quantities. Essential oils act as natural preservatives but home-made preparations will not stay fresh for long. Keep cool and preferably chilled.

❧ Apply a little of each ingredient to your skin before mixing. If your skin has an adverse reaction to any of the ingredients, don't use it.

❧ Always dilute essential oils in a vegetable carrier oil (such as sweet almond or grapeseed) before applying them to the skin.

❧ When choosing essential oils, be guided by the perfumes you find most appealing. If you don't like the smell of camomile consider using geranium instead. Pleasure is a vital part of the cleansing ritual.

❧ The recipes give suggestions for using and combining various herbs and essential oils. Once you get into the swing of it, mix and match your own using the following chart for guidance to create the perfect preparation for your skin.

❧ At the back of the book you will find a list of recommended suppliers for the ingredients you will need. Most are available by mail order. Your local healthfood store or chemist should stock certain products, too.

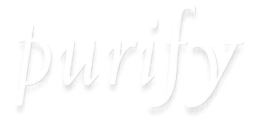

WORK WITH YOUR SKIN

Try to put together the kind of cleansing ritual that suits your own skin's needs. Bear in mind that your skin may become drier or oilier at particular times of the year. Subtle changes in its nature may even occur during the monthly cycle. If you make your own cleansers you can adapt the basic recipe formulae to suit your skin's changing needs from day to day depending on which plant extracts you use. When you don't have the time to do it yourself, seek out products containing similar pure ingredients.

Here is a guide to choosing and combining various cleansing preparations to suit different types of skin. Use this as a basic blueprint. It is essential to tune in to what works best for you and go with the flow. For recipes, see pages 20–1.

Preserving the balance – for normal skin
am – Rose Scented Milk or Geranium Skin Fresh Lotion.

pm – Jasmine Cool Cleansing Milk washed away with rose soap.

Deep cleansing – for oily skin
am – Lemon/Grapefruit Skin Fresh Lotion or lavender soap.

pm – Mint and Yarrow Cool Cleansing Milk washed away with lavender or peppermint soap.

Soft option – for dry skin
am – Elderflower/Camomile Scented Milk.

pm – Geranium and Meadowsweet Whipped Cleansing Cream wiped away with Geranium/Camomile Skin Fresh Lotion.

Soothing solutions – for sensitive skin
am – Rose/Marshmallow Scented Milk.

pm – Sandalwood and Marshmallow Whipped Cleansing Cream (or Cool Cleansing Milk if preferred), followed by Rose Skin Fresh Lotion.

— Recipes —

SKIN FRESH LOTION

30g (1oz) soapwort root
570ml (1 pint) pure spring water
4–6 drops essential oil (see below)

Rose – For normal and sensitive skin, add 4–6 drops of rose essential oil.

Lemon or grapefruit – For oily skin, add 4–6 drops of lemon or grapefruit essential oil.

Geranium – For normal skin, add 4–6 drops of geranium essential oil.

Camomile – For dry skin, add 4–6 drops of camomile essential oil.

Steep the soapwort root in water in a saucepan for 20 minutes, then heat gently and simmer for a further 20 minutes. Remove from the heat, strain and add the essential oils when cool. Pour into a bottle and keep chilled. Keeps fresh for up to 4 days.

COOL CLEANSING MILK

$1/2$ teaspoon cocoa butter
1 teaspoon white beeswax
1 teaspoon emulsifying wax
3 tablespoons cold-pressed oil – sunflower or sweet almond

4 tablespoons herbal infusion (see below)
4–6 drops essential oil (see below)
1 tablespoon pure spring water

Jasmine – For normal skin, use jasmine flowers for infusion and scent with jasmine essential oil.

Mint and yarrow – For oily skin, use yarrow herb for infusion and scent with peppermint essential oil.

Sandalwood and marshmallow – For sensitive skin, use marshmallow root for infusion and scent with sandalwood essential oil.

Melt the cocoa butter, beeswax and emulsifying wax in a glass bowl placed over a saucepan containing a small quantity of boiling water (like a bain marie). When they turn liquid, slowly drip in the oil while stirring with a wooden spoon. Mix thoroughly and then gradually stir in the herbal infusion. Remove the bowl from the heat and allow the mixture to cool, stirring occasionally. When lukewarm, add the essential oils and mix well. Now stir in about a tablespoon of pure spring water, a little at a time, until the cream becomes milky. Keeps fresh for 1 week when chilled.

SCENTED MILKS

1 tablespoon dried flowers or herbs (see below)
280ml ($^1/_2$ pint) fresh organic milk

Rose – For normal and sensitive skin, use
1 tablespoon of dried rose petals.
Elderflower or camomile – For dry skin, use
1 tablespoon of dried elderflowers or
camomile flowers.
Marshmallow – For sensitive skin, use 1 tablespoon of marshmallow root.

Steep the flowers or herbs in the cold milk in a
saucepan for 1 hour, then warm gently for about
10 minutes. Leave to cool, then strain. You can
now add a drop or two of sweet-smelling
essential oil like rose, jasmine or ylang ylang, if
desired. When chilled, it will keep fresh for 4
days. Throw away any left-over cleanser and
make another batch.

WHIPPED CLEANSING CREAM

1 teaspoon cocoa butter
1 teaspoon white beeswax
1 teaspoon emulsifying wax
2 tablespoons organic sunflower oil
2 tablespoons herbal infusion (see below)
4–6 drops essential oil (see below)

Geranium and meadowsweet – For dry skin,
use meadowsweet for infusion and scent with
geranium essential oil.
Sandalwood and marshmallow – For sensitive
skin, use marshmallow root for infusion and
scent with sandalwood essential oil.

Melt the cocoa butter, beeswax and emulsifying wax in a glass bowl placed over a saucepan
containing a small quantity of boiling water.
When they turn liquid, slowly drip in the oil,
stirring all the time with a wooden spoon.
Gradually add in the herbal infusion. Remove
the bowl from the saucepan and allow to cool,
stirring occasionally. When lukewarm, drop in
the essential oil and blend well. Pour into a
glass jar. Keeps fresh for 1 week when chilled.

For information on how to make an infusion,
see page 187.

Refreshing – The Finishing Touch

Light floral tonics that cool and refresh the skin
have a double role to play.

Firstly, they remove any traces of cleanser that may have been left behind, at the same time helping to tighten the pores which makes them look smaller and more refined. Secondly, they plump up the skin cells with a fine layer of moisture which can be sealed in by applying your day- or night-cream. This helps to keep skin looking fresh and feeling soft for longer.

The gentlest refreshers are essentially water that's been infused with plant extracts. Many commercial toners contain around 70 per cent alcohol which imparts a fresh, tingling sensation to the skin. Although it is good at cutting through oil, alcohol can irritate and dehydrate the skin. There are gentler plant astringents to choose from such as witch hazel and lavender which help to rebalance the activity of the oil-producing glands.

FLORAL WATERS

When essential oils are extracted by a process of distillation from an infusion of flower petals, the left-over liquid is known as floral water. Many make wonderful skin refiners.

Rose water ~ Although the perfume is somewhat muted, rose water still retains a hint of rose essence as well as many of the petals' skin-softening qualities. Alternatively you can make your own version by suspending a few drops of pure rose otto essential oil in a teaspoon of clear alcohol (such as vodka) and dissolving this in a cup of pre-boiled pure spring water.

Rose water makes a lovely tonic for most skin types, especially those with a tendency towards dryness and sensitivity. It is an invaluable ingredient for moisturisers, masks and other preparations.

Orange flower water ~ This sweet-smelling water is left behind when neroli essential oil is extracted from an infusion of orange flower blossoms. Genuine orange flower water is known as a 'hydrolat' and is only available from aromatherapy suppliers. In France orange flower water is diluted with hot water and sweetened with honey to make a soothing bedtime drink. Marie Antoinette is famed for using orange flower water to brighten her sallow complexion.

Make your own by suspending a few drops of pure neroli essential oil in a teaspoon of clear alcohol and then dissolving in a cup of pre-boiled pure spring water.

Orange flower water is slightly more astringent than rose water which makes it a good tonic for oily and dull complexions. It can be added to creams and masks specifically designed for this type of skin.

Lavender flower water ~ A by-product of the distillation of lavender essential oil, this water was once highly valued as a cologne. Like the essential oil, it has a wonderfully soothing and uplifting aroma. On the skin it brings clarity to sallow, oily and blemished complexions as well as encouraging healing.

Again it makes a superb addition to cosmetic preparations for slightly troubled skin.

Witch hazel ~ This lotion comes from a small, twisted tree that is native to North America. Native American tribes traditionally used decoctions of the bark in poultices to reduce swelling and inflammation. Distilled witch hazel contains the steam-distilled active constituents of the leaves and twigs preserved in alcohol. It is a well-known first-aid remedy for treating cuts, bruises and swelling.

FLOWER REFRESHER
(for all skin types)

Combine equal amounts of rose water, orange flower water and lavender water and pour into a spritzer bottle or atomiser. (30ml or 2 tablespoons of each makes enough to last up to 1 month.) Spray the face after cleansing.

LEMON ZEST REFRESHER

Leaves oily skin squeaky clean and restores the acid mantle.

570ml (1 pint) boiled pure spring water
1 teaspoon fresh lemon juice
4 teaspoons vegetable glyercine
2 drops rose and 2 drops camomile essential oils

Add all the ingredients together in a capped bottle, shake well to blend and decant into a spritzer bottle. Spray after cleansing. Keeps fresh for 1 week when chilled.

Being astringent and mildly antiseptic, witch hazel makes a good refreshing lotion for treating oily skin and pimples, as well as refining enlarged pores.

You can either use the floral waters singly or in combination as a refresher.

Buffed to Perfection

Exfoliation involves buffing away any dull flaky cells from the skin's surface to reveal a more perfect complexion.

Regular sloughing not only keeps skin looking fresh and feeling super-soft, it also keeps the pores clear which prevents the clogging that causes blackheads and spots. As oil flows freely to the surface to form its moisture-resistant film, even dry skin benefits from this kind of treatment.

POLISHED PERFECTION

Creams and pastes infused with gritty, skin-buffing particles are known as physical exfoliators or skin scrubs. They certainly do the trick, but if the grains are too abrasive they can actually leave scratch marks on the skin's surface.

Many cosmetic companies now use tiny spherical beads designed to glide over the skin surface so they polish without doing such damage. Nature also boasts some softer options to the once popular ground-nut kernels. Finely milled almonds and oatmeal have a gentle, sloughing action and are also known for their skin-softening and nourishing properties.

§ Pineapple or papaya fruits contain protein-digesting enzymes (bromelain and papain) which dissolve away cellular debris and loosen dead cells clinging tenaciously to the skin's surface. Try the **Pineapple or Papaya Peel** opposite.

FRUIT REFINERS

Fruit acids or alpha-hydroxy acids (AHAs) exfoliate by dissolving the glue that holds dead skin cells together. While fruit acids such as glycolic acid occur naturally in sugar cane, citrus fruits, grapes, milk and wine, AHAs in commercial skin creams are often made in the laboratory. Preparations containing weak dilutions of fruit acids ensure old cells are shed evenly and swiftly. This keeps the skin looking fresh and radiant. At higher concentrations they form the basis of professional skin peels that strip away the stratum corneum to expose fresher, more youthful-looking epidermal cells beneath. But if the protective layer is slowly eroded away, skin becomes more vulnerable to sun and other environmental damage. AHAs therefore have the potential to encourage sensitivity. Use these products wisely and moderately. Once daily will keep your skin looking fresh and bright.

— Recipes —

EXFOLIATING CREAM BASE

1 teaspoon cocoa butter

1 teaspoon white beeswax

1 teaspoon emulsifying wax

2 tablespoons organic sunflower oil

2 tablespoons pure spring water

Melt the cocoa butter, beeswax and emulsifying wax in a glass bowl placed over a saucepan containing a small quantity of boiling water. When they are liquid, slowly drip the oil into the mix stirring all the time with a wooden spoon. Then gradually stir in the water. Remove the bowl from the saucepan and allow to cool, stirring occasionally. This is your base cream. The recipe makes enough to last about 2 weeks. Keep it in the fridge but leave out at room temperature for 1–2 hours before using.

ALMOND REFINING CREAM

Add 1 teaspoon of finely ground almonds to 1 teaspoon of your base cream and blend. Massage gently into the skin reaching into every corner and then sweep away with a warm, damp muslin cloth. Spray with the refresher of your choice (see pages 22–3).

PINEAPPLE OR PAPAYA PEEL

Add 1 teaspoon of freshly squeezed pineapple or papaya juice to 1 teaspoon of your base cream and blend. Massage into the skin, especially around the base of the nose and under the jawline. Leave for a few minutes or until it begins to tingle and then remove with a warm, damp muslin cloth. Spray with your refresher (see pages 22–3).

LAVENDER AND ALMOND BODY POLISHER

1 tablespoon finely ground oatmeal

1 tablespoon finely ground almonds

$^1/_2$ tablespoon kaolin (see page 182)

1 tablespoon hot boiled pure spring water

1 tablespoon aloe vera juice

$^1/_2$ tablespoon sweet almond oil

4 drops lavender essential oil

Spoon the oatmeal, ground almonds and kaolin into a small bowl. Slowly stir in the water, aloe vera juice and finally the sweet almond oil. When lukewarm and thickening, stir in the lavender essential oil. Rub over the body, concentrating on rough areas such as the elbows, knees and soles of the feet. Rinse off with warm water.

Deep Cleansing

Cleansing can be taken one step further with treatments that harness
the skin-purifying powers of various types of clay and mud.

PORCELAIN FINISH

The clarifying properties of clay have been
recognised for centuries. Each type of clay has a
slightly different effect on the skin depending on
its composition of minerals and plant-derived
nutrients. Yet all share the same remarkable
powers of absorption.

Every clay particle carries a slight negative
charge and, like a magnet, attracts the positively
charged impurities found both on the surface of
the skin and within the body. Applied to the
skin, clay literally vacuums stale oil and cellular
debris from the pores. This oil and debris is
responsible for blackheads and creates conditions conducive to spots. These earthy powders
form the basis of many professional face and
body masks.

The clays most frequently used in deep-
cleansing masks are kaolin, green clay and fuller's
earth. Green clay has healing and slightly antiseptic qualities which makes it useful for treating
congested and problem skins. It has a rebalancing action so helping to normalise an oily skin
while softening and revitalising a dry one.

Fuller's earth is so effective at absorbing toxins
and impurities that it is used to treat the victims
of radiation exposure.

Ingredients such as honey, oils and essential
oils can be added to these clays to make masks
that are tailored to your skin's particular needs.

GLORIOUS MUD

Mud packs are a popular deep-cleansing treatment. Many of the oldest spas around the world
were established at places renowned for their
unique therapeutic muds. These include the
'fango' found at certain natural springs in Italy,
the mineral-rich mud collected from the Dead
Sea, and moor, a peat rich in healing herbs and
plants from Austria (see also Chapter 12).

Mud masks also generate an inner warmth
that promotes perspiration. As toxins are drawn
out through the skin, they become absorbed by
the drying mud.

These muds are sometimes blended with oils
and plant essences to make a warm paste which
is then smeared over the skin. The body is
usually wrapped in foil or a sort of clingfilm to

— A clean sweep —

§ Wiping away your cleansing milk or cream with a finely textured muslin cloth may provide all the buffing a dry or sensitive skin needs.

§ For the gentlest exfoliation of all try smearing a teaspoon of clear honey over your face, then patting lightly and rapidly with the fingertips all over your face for about 5 minutes. The old cells stick to the honey and patting lifts them away while helping to plump up the cells underneath. Rinse off with warm water and pat dry, then spray with the refresher of your choice (see pages 22–3).

seal in the heat and promote sweating. These kind of treatments may be done at home. They are messy, however, and you may need a little assistance and a shower close at hand.

SPUN STRAWBERRY MASK
(for normal to dry skins)

1 tablespoon kaolin
1 tablespoon clear honey
1 tablespoon natural yoghurt
4 fresh strawberries, sliced

Put all the ingredients in a blender and whizz into a rich pink cream. Apply to the face and neck, place cottonwool pads soaked in rose water over the eyes, and leave for 15 minutes. Rinse off and spray with the refresher of your choice (see pages 22–3).

PEPPERMINT PURIFYING MASK
(for oily and congested skins)

1 tablespoon fuller's earth or green clay
2 tablespoons peppermint infusion (place a peppermint tea bag in a cup of boiling water for 5 minutes)
1 tablespoon aloe vera juice
1–2 drops tea tree essential oil

Spoon the fuller's earth or green clay into a small china bowl and slowly stir in the peppermint infusion and aloe vera juice to make a thick paste. Drop in the tea tree essential oil and mix again. Apply a fine layer to the skin and a double layer to areas prone to congestion, such as the oily central panel and chin. Leave for 10 minutes or until the mask starts to dry, then rinse off and spray with the refresher of your choice (see pages 22–3).

Cleansing from Within

To keep skin looking fresh and clear, a good cleansing regime goes
hand in hand with steps that preserve inner purity.

Nowadays our bodies are increasingly bombarded with pollutants and chemicals which overwhelm its natural coping systems. Accumulating toxins underlie many skin complaints and clearing them from the body can work wonders for restoring the natural clarity that comes from deep within.

WHAT ARE TOXINS?

Toxin is an umbrella term that describes any substance or chemical that interferes with normal metabolism. They can be ordinary metabolic wastes, viruses and bacteria, synthetic chemicals such as pesticide residues, and natural chemicals found in foods and drinks such as caffeine and alcohol. Like rubbish, toxins clog up the system and interfere with the smooth functioning of our organs and tissues, so we must get rid of them.

PATHWAYS TO PURITY

There are several paths for toxin elimination and ensuring that these channels are working smoothly and efficiently is the key to inner cleanliness. Skin itself is an organ of elimination

so if the other paths are congested it may take the strain. Puffiness and spots are a tell-tale sign that it's time to detox.

Blood and lymph ~ These are responsible for picking up toxins from the tissues and taking them to the liver. Tension, lack of exercise and anything else that impedes good circulation can result in wastes collecting in certain areas of the body.

To purify, take regular exercise, practise body brushing, eat plenty of cabbage, garlic, onions, beetroot, blackberries and blueberries. Wheatgrass juice is a supreme blood and lymph cleanser (see pages 197–9 for suppliers).

The liver ~ This is the body's major cleansing organ. It neutralises poisons and wastes as well as building essential molecules. Eating lots of fatty food and drinking too much alcohol taxes this organ. Waves of nausea, early morning tiredness and lack of appetite are tell-tale signs of an overburdened liver. Pent-up emotions like anger and frustration also interfere with its work.

To purify, eat lots of bitter foods such as grapefruit, lemon, endive and dandelion leaves. Extra-virgin olive oil, garlic, ginger, cabbage, artichokes and milk thistle herb (*Silybum marianum* – often abbreviated to silymarin) are especially renowned for their liver-cleansing and fortifying qualities.

The kidneys ~ These are filtering systems where wastes are removed from the blood, diluted with water and flushed away. Eating salt-laden food encourages the kidneys to reabsorb too much water which may lead to fluid retention and puffy looking skin. Coffee, alcohol and diuretics on the other hand encourage excessive water loss and can cause mild dehydration. Dark circles and bags under the eyes are signs of poorly functioning kidneys.

To purify, drink plenty of pure spring water and cut back on salty foods. Good kidney toning and cleansing foods include artichokes, celery and asparagus. Sip infusions of tonic herbs like goldenrod, fennel and uva ursi. Add parsley, another kidney tonic, to salads and cooked dishes. Drinking home-made barley water is a great way to cleanse and soothe the kidneys.

The large intestine ~ This clears digested food remains from the body. Rhythmic contractions known as peristalsis move the waste material along the colon. As stress and tension interfere with these contractions and upset the natural flow of wastes, both diarrhoea and constipation can result. Over time the sticky remains of refined foods such as white bread and pasta may cling to the intestinal walls and clog up the system.

To purify, the natural roughage in wholegrain foods, fresh vegetables and fruits acts as an intestinal broom and ensures the swift passage of wastes through the colon. Soluble fibres like pectin (in apple skins) and alginin (in seaweed) mop up toxic substances and ensure they get removed from the body rather than reabsorbed. Psyllium husks (available from healthfood stores) work in the same way, so try adding a teaspoon to your morning cereal.

GOING GREEN

Green plants are powerful allies in the pursuit of purity. Leafy vegetables such as spinach and watercress and herbs such as parsley and comfrey are rich in chlorophyll, the green plant pigment long recognised as having powerful cleansing properties. Chlorophyll in the leaves absorbs energy from the sun and uses it for photosynthesis, a plant's equivalent of breathing. Within the body, chlorophyll helps to clear out

– Keeping clean –

- Eat at least one large green leafy salad every day.

- Choose organically produced food whenever possible.

- Avoid drinking coffee and tea when you feel stressed – opt for refreshing tisanes such as elderflower, peppermint and camomile instead. (For information on making tisanes, see page 187.)

- Try to drink a litre (1³/₄ pints) of pure spring or mineral water each day, little and often.

- Keep in tune with the seasons. Choose seasonal fruits and vegetables, eat cooling salad dishes in the summer and warm soups, broths and casseroles in the winter.

tissue wastes that can interfere with cellular metabolism and is well known for its deodorant effect. Chlorophyll also seems to strengthen the cells so they are more resilient to the corrosive effects of pollution and ultraviolet light. Both enriching your diet with chlorophyll-rich plants and applying them externally can have a remarkable effect on the texture and quality of skin. Watercress helps to heal acne, comfrey softens and smoothes, while a good splash of wheatgrass added to the bath makes a great skin cleanser.

- Rich sources of chlorophyll include spinach, kale, cabbage greens, lamb's lettuce, cos lettuce, watercress, green pepper, dandelion leaves, chlorella (see pages 57–8), spirulina (see page 57), parsley, sage, borage, comfrey, basil, sprouted alfalfa, wheat, oat and barley grasses.

Quick cleanse

For one day a week and at least once a month have nothing but water, fresh fruit and vegetable juices. This gives all the elimination systems a well-deserved rest and coaxes the toxins from the tissues. On the days before and after this mini fast eat lightly to allow your body to acclimatise to this change in routine.

Steam Cleaning

Regular steaming treatments are a wonderful way
to promote deep cleansing.

Bathing in hot vapour promotes perspiration and coaxes deep-seated wastes from the body. Steaming also encourages pores to relax and liquifies oils so they flow more freely to the surface, so clearing and preventing blackheads. Turkish steam baths are ideal for a whole body cleanse. Always shower afterwards, wrap up warmly in a towel and ideally relax for 20 minutes rather than dressing straightaway.

Remember to replace lost fluids by drinking at least a glass of pure spring water after a steam treatment.

Steaming is a good way to prepare skin for a deep-cleansing face mask or body wrap as it opens the pores and sets the elimination process in motion. There is no point trying to nourish the skin while it is busy throwing off toxins, so save these treatments for later.

Do-it-yourself steam facial

Pour boiling water into a large bowl or basin, cover your head with a towel and allow your skin to bathe in the steam for 5–10 minutes. Herbs and essential oils can be added to the water for a more individualised and rebalancing skin treatment. Finish the treatment by splashing with cool water to remove wastes from the skin's surface.

- Infuse 30g (1oz) of herb in 1 litre (1³/₄ pints) of boiling pure spring water.

- Add 1–2 drops of essential oil to 1 litre (1³/₄ pints) of just boiled pure spring water.

For a decongesting steam clean use infusions of echinacea, camomile or elderflowers, or essential oils of eucalyptus and camomile. For other recommendations see the chart on page 17.

A steam facial helps cleanse most skin types and is especially beneficial for oily complexions with blocked pores. Avoid steaming if your skin is highly sensitive, prone to broken capillaries, or if your acne flares up in hot, humid conditions.

soft

CHAPTER THREE

Moisturising

~

The Essence of Softness

Skin loves water. This essential element endows skin with youthful softness and smoothness. But biting winds, intense heat and artificially dry environments draw water from the skin. At times like these, skin needs extra protection and water-replenishing treatments to preserve perfection.

Our affinity with water is not just skin deep. Spraying, showering and bathing in fresh and sea water has the power to restore and revitalise our complexion, soothe our psyche and lift our spirits. Water works wonders, so take the plunge.

Be moisturised.

Liquid Assets

Water is the essence of life. This element makes up 75 per cent of our
body's composition, a legacy perhaps of our watery origins.

Around 9 litres (16 pints) of water are present in the skin itself. When cells in the epidermis are rich in moisture they appear plumped up, like soft and bouncy cushions. The plum and prune analogy is as old as the hills, but it conjures up a realistic image of what happens when these cells lose moisture. Skin feels tight and fine lines appear, making it look old before its time.

WATERTIGHT

Skin has been designed to preserve its precious moisture and there are various efficient barrier systems that prevent it from drying out.

Stratum corneum ~ A protective outer seal of dry, flaky cells which lie in neatly packed layers. These cells are held together with an intercellular glue made from waxy substances like ceramides and cholesterol derivatives.

Over-exposure to strong detergents and alkaline soaps erodes this glue and disrupts the structure of the stratum corneum. Over-zealous buffing with exfoliating scrubs may also damage this protective layer, as can chafing winter winds.

Hydrolipidic mantle ~ A natural moisturiser made from our own oily and watery secretions which forms a fine watertight seal over the skin's surface. The more oil your skin produces, the better lubricated it will be. While clearing away stale oils at the beginning and end of each day, the skin must also be allowed to replenish this moisturising mantle. The sebaceous glands produce less oil as we get older and by the age of fifty most skins will start to feel slightly dry unless we supplement their natural protection.

Cell membranes ~ Like every living cell in our body, the epidermal cells are surrounded by fluid membranes made mostly of essential fatty acid (EFA) molecules and cholesterol. There are two basic essential fatty acids – linoleic acid and alpha-linolenic acid – which we must get from food although they can also be absorbed into the skin. From these two EFAs others can be made. Long ago scientists noted that when these nutrients were missing from the diet, skin lost water at an alarming rate and soon became dry, flaky and itchy.

Essential fatty acids are easily damaged by exposure to the sun's ultraviolet light, toxic chemicals in cigarette smoke and environmental pollutants. They can be protected by antioxidants such as vitamins A, C and E.

UNDER SEIGE

Skin's resilience to environmental onslaughts is largely determined by the effectiveness of these barrier systems. A well-structured stratum corneum, an evenly distributed hydrolipidic layer and healthy cell membranes are your skin's best defence against the elements. But these protective barriers are not infallible and, if any of them are slightly flawed, skin will lose moisture.

A temperate climate of warm breezes and frequent rain showers poses little threat to the skin's water reserves. Spring and autumn tend to be the seasons when skin feels most comfortable. Blasts of icy winter wind can deplete the skin's

— Skin saving tip —

To protect your skin from central heating, place bowls of water scented with a few drops of essential oils around the room. Use uplifting jasmine during the day, soothing neroli at night or mind-clearing essences like lemon and peppermint in the office. The heavenly perfumed rose, sandalwood and ylang ylang oils also work well.

precious moisture reserves. For every 7–8°C (45–6°F) temperature drop below 20°C (68°F), the amount of water lost to the air doubles.

Inside central heating provides little in the way of relief as it re-creates an atmosphere as arid as the Sahara desert. Like cold, dry air, sun-parched atmospheres have a very dehydrating effect on the skin. This is where moisturisers come to the rescue.

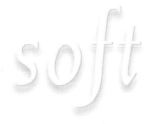

Protect and Preserve ~
The Essence of Moisturising

Moisturisers are preparations that preserve skin's natural moisture and consequently its soft, silken texture.

They work primarily by trapping moisture in the uppermost layer of the skin so it feels softer and smoother. Most moisturisers are blends of oil and water which replicate the skin's own hydrolipidic mantle. The richer creams are made by suspending droplets of water in oil while the finer milks are oil-in-water emulsions.

We tend to prefer the lighter preparations because they sink swiftly into the skin and leave no oily residues behind. Being rich in water, these preparations deliver instant softness, but dry atmospheres also take this moisture away from the skin so their benefits are usually short lived. Creams rich in oils may feel a little heavier but they provide longer-lasting protection against the elements. Other ingredients can be added to this basic oil-and-water formula to boost its moisturising power.

Moisture magnets ~ These are substances that suck up water like sponges and can help to hold moisture in the skin. Cosmetic companies favour ingredients like hyaluronic acid and sodium PCA but vegetable glycerine is a pure plant-derived alternative that works well too.

Super-saturates ~ Aloe vera comes from the leaves of a cactus which inhabits arid landscapes. As well as having amazing powers for absorbing and retaining moisture, aloe has soothing, anti-inflammatory and healing properties. Using neat aloe vera juice or gel is like giving your skin a refreshing drink. It can also be blended into creams to create light but highly effective moisturisers.

Inner strength ~ Essential fatty acids can be taken up by the skin and used to strengthen and rebuild the membranes that hold moisture in the cells. Some of the richest plant sources are flax, hemp, evening primrose, borage, walnut and sunflower seed oil. As essential fatty molecules are easily destroyed by heat, light and exposure to air, they must be kept in tinted bottles and stored in a dark cool place. Adding a little vitamin E to these oils also acts as a natural preservative.

Plant power ~ Many herbs are rich in softening substances. Comfrey is rich in allantoin which is renowned for its skin-enhancing qualities. The best moisturisers are made with infusions of herbs like comfrey, marshmallow, elderflower and lime blossom.

HOW MUCH, HOW OFTEN?

There are no hard and fast rules about moisturising. If your skin is healthy and cleansed kindly, its own protective barrier may require very little extra assistance when the temperature is mild and the air rich in moisture. Remember oily secretions diminish with age and skin may require more moisturising as time goes by. Changes in the seasons and going on holiday to countries with hot, dry climates may increase your skin's need for protection. A fluid formulation that disappears into the skin may be fine for the summer, but you may need a creamier, more protective preparation during the cold winter months. As the face and hands are exposed to the elements virtually all the time they are likely to need more moisturising than skin on other areas of the body.

Let your own skin be your guide. Providing it feels soft there is no need to slather on moisturising cream morning, noon and night.

— Some things you should know —

- Fine skin is more susceptible to dryness and fine lines. With age the skin becomes thinner as cell renewal slows down, so you may need a richer moisturiser as you get older.
- The skin around the eyes is particularly thin and delicate. The richer, heavier creams may encourage puffiness in this area, especially if worn during the night. So, opt for light gel formulations packed with protective antioxidant nutrients and moisture magnets.
- Lips have no protective oily secretions of their own and will need the added lubrication of waxy balms, especially during summer and winter.
- As our hands are washed many times a day and are out in all weathers, they need the extra protection of rich, creamy moisturisers. Apply frequently in the winter months.
- Jet travel is incredibly dehydrating. Pop a small tub of aloe vera gel scented with a few drops of lavender into your hand luggage and apply a little every 30 minutes to keep your skin feeling cool and fresh.

— Recipes —

The beauty of making your own moisturisers is that by playing around with the proportions of oil and water you will hit upon the consistency that best suits your skin. **Rose Petal Moisturiser** (see below) is light yet protective and is designed to suit most skin types.

ROSE PETAL MOISTURISER

1 teaspoon white beeswax
1 teaspoon cocoa butter
1 teaspoon emulsifying wax
1 tablespoon sweet almond oil, preferably organic
1 tablespoon rose water
1 tablespoon herb infusion
1 capsule vitamin E oil
1 capsule or $^1/_2$ teaspoon evening primrose or borage oil
1 teaspoon vegetable glycerine
1 tablespoon aloe vera gel
6 drops rose essential oil

Melt the beeswax, cocoa butter and emulsifying wax in a glass bowl over a saucepan of boiling water. Slowly pour in the almond oil, drop by drop, stirring continuously with a wooden spoon and then slowly add in the rose water and herbal infusion. Remove the bowl from the heat. Next, pierce the vitamin E capsule with a pin and squeeze the oil into the bowl. Stir in along with the evening primrose or borage oil and the vegetable glycerine.

Allow to cool, stirring occasionally. When the mixture is lukewarm, blend in the aloe vera gel a little at a time. Finally add your essential oil. Store in a tinted glass jar and keep cool. Keeps fresh for up to 4 weeks.

❧ Rose smells wonderful and suits most skins but, if you love the aroma of lavender, using essential oil of lavender to scent your moisturiser will really lift your spirits. Follow your instincts.

ROSE AND ALOE EYE GEL

1 tablespoon aloe vera gel
15 drops carrot oil
15 drops evening primrose oil
1 capsule vitamin E oil
2 drops rose essential oil

Spoon the aloe vera gel into a small bowl (a ramekin is perfect) and drop in all the other ingredients. Stir to blend the ingredients together and spoon into a small glass jar. Keep chilled. Lasts for 4 weeks.

JASMINE SKIN DRINK

$^1/_2$–1 teaspoon cocoa butter

1 teaspoon white beeswax

1 teaspoon emulsifying wax

3 tablespoons sweet almond oil

3 tablespoons pure spring water

1 tablespoon aloe vera gel

1 capsule vitamin E oil

4 drops jasmine essential oil

2 drops ylang ylang essential oil

Melt the cocoa butter, beeswax and emulsifying wax in a glass bowl over a saucepan of boiling water. When liquid, gradually stir in the sweet almond oil with a wooden spoon. When blended slowly stir in the spring water. It should form a thin white emulsion. Remove the bowl from the heat, pierce the vitamin E capsule and add the oil droplets. Allow to cool, stirring from time to time. When lukewarm, blend in the aloe vera gel a little at a time, then add in the essential oils.

Pour into a large-necked glass bottle and keep cool. Keeps fresh for up to 4 weeks.

MINTY LIPS

1 teaspoon white beeswax

3 teaspoons jojoba oil

1 teaspoon carrot oil

1 capsule of vitamin E oil

5 drops St John's wort tincture

$^1/_2$ teaspoon clear honey

2 drops peppermint essential oil

Melt the beeswax in a glass bowl over a saucepan of boiling water. Slowly add in the jojoba and carrot oils, stirring all the time. Remove the bowl from the heat. Pierce the vitamin E capsule and squeeze in the oil, then drop in the St John's wort tincture. When cool, stir in the honey and add the peppermint essential oil.

Spoon this golden balm into a small glass jar and use sparingly. Keeps fresh for up to 4 weeks.

– *Tips* –

On hot sunny days carry a bottle of pure spring or mineral water with you to sip to prevent dehydration.

Landing in a hot country after a long-haul flight is seriously dehydrating, so be extra careful to drink plenty of water both during and after the flight.

The Beauty of Water

Water is skin's most essential nutrient. Plentiful supplies of this crystal-clear liquid replenish moisture from deep within.

Water is also nature's most effective internal cleanser for it dissolves away wastes to preserve skin's clarity and freshness from the inside out. But how much water do we need to keep our skin looking its best?

FLUID LEVEL

We can live without food for several days, even weeks, but if deprived of water for more than a day or two we could not survive. Each day our body loses fluid in the form of perspiration and this needs to be replenished. When the humidity level is normal, at between 40–60 per cent we can lose anything up to a litre ($1\frac{1}{4}$ pints) of fluid in just 12 hours, even when it's chilly. This means drinking at least 1 and preferably 2 litres ($3\frac{1}{2}$ pints) of pure water every single day.

In parched environments we lose body fluids much more rapidly. Heat makes matters worse for when the temperature soars our sweat glands work overtime to keep us cool. The more fluid your body loses, the more water you need to drink to keep levels topped up. Feeling thirsty is a sign that your body is slightly dehydrated and needs more water. When dehydration rises to around 4 per cent we can feel tired, impatient, headachy and slightly nauseous. The mid-afternoon energy dip can often be relieved quite simply by drinking a long glass of cool, sparkling H_2O.

Strenuous activity also increases water loss. While it's good to sweat out unwanted wastes, we can lose up to a litre ($1\frac{3}{4}$ pints) of fluid during an hour of aerobic exercise. The fitter you are, the more you lose as your body becomes adept at cooling down. It is important to compensate for this water loss.

Emotions such as anxiety, fear, embarrassment and sexual excitement also spur the sweat glands into action which means we often feel thirstier in times of stress.

FINELY BALANCED

Fluid balance is a complex affair and various factors encourage tissues to retain fluid or promote diuresis (water loss). Among these are certain hormones. Fluctuating levels of oestrogen, a key menstrual hormone, in the days leading up to a period often cause water reten-

40

tion and bloating. Stress and long-distance travel upset hormone balance in ways that make you feel thirsty and waterlogged at the same time.

Dietary factors may also upset the equilibrium. Foods rich in sodium or salt encourage water retention because salt attracts water and vice versa. As perspiration contains salt as well as water, excessive sweating may deplete both. Symptoms of sodium loss are similar to dehydration and include nausea, dizziness, vomiting, cramps, exhaustion and apathy. In hot weather and after taking vigorous exercise or having frequent saunas it may be a good idea to sprinkle a little sea salt over your food.

The mineral potassium, present within every body cell, works alongside sodium to maintain fluid balance. The kidneys keep the potassium level within certain limits but their job is harder when our diet provides much more sodium than potassium. Our early ancestors who lived entirely on unprocessed foods may have enjoyed a diet which contained much more potassium than sodium. Today the balance is firmly biased in favour of sodium. Some diuretics also flush potassium from the body. Low levels of potassium cause tissue swelling along with fatigue, weakness and headaches.

§ To keep these minerals perfectly balanced, eat plenty of potassium-rich fruits and vegetables, wholegrain cereals and avoid eating foods laden with extra salt like crisps, salted nuts and most processed foods.

§ Eat foods that gently flush away excess fluids: celery, celeriac, asparagus, artichoke, watermelon, cucumber and beetroot.

— Well-watered —

§ Begin the day with a glass of water — it helps the kidneys work well and cleanses from within.

§ Drink a glass of water at bedtime — your body loses water as you sleep.

§ Take sips of water regularly throughout the day rather than all in one go.

§ When exercising drink two glasses of water for every pound (0.5 kg) you lose through sweating.

§ Don't rely on coffee and alcohol to quench your thirst. They act as diuretics and so increase loss of fluids.

§ Sweet fizzy drinks are poor substitutes for pure water — the high sugar content actually increases thirst.

Healing Waters

When we splash, spray and bathe our bodies in water, amazing things
begin to happen.

The ancient Greeks recognised the healing power of water. At spas around the world water is used in different ways to unleash skin's natural vitality and revitalise our whole being – mind, body and spirit. The basic elements of water or hydrotherapy should be a part of your daily skincare regime.

MOTHER NATURE

We have a deep affinity with water and are captivated by thundering waterfalls, gurgling streams and reflective lakes. Simply being near water uplifts the spirit and soothes the psyche. In many cultures, water symbolises the mother. A watery environment seems to provide the comfort, security and privacy we crave when life is fraught and demanding. Being close to or enveloped in water may kindle subconscious memories of life within the womb. There's nothing quite as relaxing and liberating as floating in water. And from inner stillness and tranquillity spring renewed energy and vitality.

Natural waters that gush from the earth's inner core are renowned for their healing properties. Prized for their purity, these spring and mineral waters contain numerous health-enhancing minerals. At health spas established at these sources, the use of water to relax and revitalise the body has been perfected to a fine art. Water therapy can work wonders for restoring vitality and cultivating skin's natural beauty. Discover their benefits for yourself.

Spa treats

Hot and cold showering ~ A shower is a superb energiser. Gushing water releases negative ions into the air which make us feel calm yet refreshed. In contrast, polluted air is rich in positive ions.

Alternating hot (36.7–40°C/98–104°F) and cold (12.7–18.3°C/55–65°F) water stimulates the circulation and leaves skin glowing. Switching from warm to cold invigorates and fortifies the system, helping to boost resistance to illness.

- Always begin with a comfortably hot shower and once warmed up, switch the temperature to cold for 30–60 seconds, then turn back to warm. If you finish with a cold blast be sure to wrap up in a warm towel afterwards. After alternate showering rest for at least 5 minutes, preferably longer, before dressing.

Hot and cold foot baths are a good substitute for whole body showering.

Jet massage (douche au jet) ~ At spas powerful jets of warm (36.7–40°C/ 98–104°F) water are directed at the body from a distance. They are used to massage specific areas such as the thighs, calves, bottom and tummy to improve skin tone and refine the body contours. Blasts of water help to unearth and clear toxins from the tissues. They boost the circulation of blood and lymph.

§ At home use the shower attachment to spray your body. Work up the calves and thighs, use circular movements over the bottom and tummy. Gently spraying the breasts with chilly water on a regular basis is reputed to keep them firm and well-toned.

– Spa tips –

Drink plenty of pure spring or mineral water after showering and bathing.

Don't soak in the bath for more than 20 minutes, especially if your skin tends to be dry.

Avoid bubble baths – they are based on detergents and invariably contain artificial colours and fragrances which can irritate the skin.

Bain bouillant (bubbling bath) ~ These are deep jacuzzi-style baths fitted with underwater jets. The water constantly bubbles while the finer jets massage the body from top to toe. Herbs and essential oils may be added to the bath to enhance the benefits.

§ At home, buy fresh herbs and place a good handful in a muslin bag. Hang the bag on your bath tap, allowing the running water to flow over it and to enable the herbs to steep in the bath.

Invigorating ~ rosemary, peppermint, pine.

Relaxing ~ camomile, lavender, lime blossom, lady's mantle.

Moisturising ~ marshmallow, elderflowers, rose petals.

Fortifying ~ eucalyptus, thyme, basil.

Scented baths ~ For a luxurious perfumed bath add essential oils – either alone or chosen to complement your choice of herbs. To disperse in the water first dissolve the oil droplets (6–10) in a tablespoon of milk, preferably organic.

Deep Sea Treatments

'The sea provides a cure for all man's ills', proclaimed Euripides,
the classical Greek dramatist, nearly two millennia ago.

It certainly does wonders for our skin. Sea water purifies and nourishes, soothes and heals. Simply bathing in the sea can improve a variety of skin conditions from eczema and psoriasis to pimples and puffiness. What makes this salty solution so special?

MARINE MAGIC

Back in the early 1900s, a French doctor called René Quinton showed that live human cells soaked in sea water not only stayed alive, they also thrived. Sea water is not just a solution of salt. In composition it is uncannily similar to our own blood plasma and contains traces of essential minerals such as calcium, potassium, sodium, iron and zinc, plus a wealth of trace elements and organic substances.

Thalassotherapy (sea water) experts believe these marine elements may be taken up by the skin through osmosis and reach the bloodstream where they help to restore and preserve good health. But for optimal absorption the sea water should be warmed, preferably to around body temperature.

Thalassotherapy or sea water therapy is similar to other hydrotherapy treatments but filtered and warmed sea water is used in place of spring water. Thalassotherapy is harder to bring into the bathroom, so next time you are by the sea make the most of it.

- Wallow in the warmer, shallow pools.
- Stand thigh-deep in breaking waves for a stimulating massage.
- Wade through the water to firm up the muscles in the lower body, and take long, deep breaths of revitalising sea air.

WONDER WEED

Seaweed harvested from the purest marine waters is an integral part of thalassotherapy. This slippery sea vegetable is valued for an ability to promote weight loss, encourage deep cleansing, boost blood circulation and lymphatic drainage, and soothe muscular aches and pains. It is used to treat a variety of skin problems from dryness and acne to cellulite.

– Sea bathing –

Soaking in salt water has many benefits. It cleanses the skin, promotes detoxification and is said to cleanse the aura. As well as having mild anti-bacterial properties, a sea soak also soothes away aches and pains. Afterwards skin feels wonderfully refreshed and silky smooth.

- Toss a good handful of sea salt into your bath while the hot water is running and soak for up to 20 minutes.

- An Epsom salt bath promotes perspiration and helps to flush out toxins as well as relieving bodily aches.

- Dead Sea salts are renowned for their skin-healing properties. The Dead Sea is unique and boasts mineral concentrations ten times greater than ordinary sea water. The salts are especially rich in bromide which may explain its relaxing effect. Bathing in the Dead Sea combined with mud masks and controlled sunbathing can work wonders for dry, itchy skin conditions, most notably psoriasis. You will need to add about 2kg (4lbs) of Dead Sea salt to a hot bath (25°C/77°F) and soak for 10–20 minutes (no longer) to re-create the full benefits.

- Try a salty scrub. Shake a little sea salt into a tablespoon of olive oil and rub all over the body before bathing. Concentrate on rough areas such as the elbows, knees and soles of the feet. This leaves skin smooth, soft and glowing.

Seaweed treats

While there are some benefits to collecting seaweed from the beach, rubbing it into your body and hanging it in the bath, you will get better results from using the professionally prepared variety. For spa treatments, the seaweed cells are exploded by ultrasound to release the active ingredients and then pulverised to form a powder. The skin then draws from the seaweed the vitamins, minerals and trace elements it needs for optimum health.

- 'Enveloppement d'algues' or seaweed mask is a popular spa treatment. Warm seaweed paste is smeared over the skin from neck to toes, then your body is wrapped first in clingfilm and then in foil to seal in the heat. Warmth encourages the uptake of seaweed nutrients into the skin and encourages the elimination of wastes.

— Recipes —

SEAWEED BODY WRAP

175g (6oz) seaweed powder
2 drops lavender or rosemary essential oil
30ml (2 tablespoons) sweet almond or grape-
    seed oil

Mix the seaweed powder with a little warm
water to moisten it. Add the essential oil to the
vegetable oil and then stir into the seaweed
powder to make a thick paste. Add a little
more water until you achieve the right consistency for smearing over the skin. For best
results exfoliate the skin and have a warm
shower or bath first. Apply the paste all over
the body, starting with the feet. (It's incredibly
messy so have plenty of sponges and towels
handy.) If possible, wrap your body in foil or
clingfilm (you will need some assistance) and
relax for 20–30 minutes before showering off.

SEAWEED BATH

$^1/_2$ cup seaweed powder
2–3 drops lavender or rosemary essential oil

Add the seaweed powder to your bath as it is
running and soak for 20 minutes. To mask the
rather fishy aroma add a few drops of sweet-
smelling lavender or rosemary essential oil as
well. Have a good shower before wrapping up
warmly in a towel and lying down for 10–15
minutes.

soft

vitality

CHAPTER FOUR

Nourishing

~

The Essence of Vitality

Skin thrives on foods brimming with natural goodness, for nutrients are the building blocks of perfect skin. From age-retarding antioxidants present in brightly coloured fruits and vegetables to energising vitamins in cereals, nuts and seeds, each nutrient has a special role to play in keeping our skin healthy and vibrant. Common skin problems are a sign that certain essential nutrients may be in short supply. Nothing revitalises the skin quite like fresh, wholesome food, so indulge yourself.

Be nourished.

Food for Thought

The average life of a skin cell is about 28 days. As old cells reach the
end of their days, new ones are forming to take their place. A spectrum
of different nutrients are needed to create and nurture these new cells.

To ensure our skin reaches its potential for perfection it is important to choose foods that supply all these essential skin ingredients. If our diet is lacking, skin is the first to give it away.

Dry skin may be gasping for essential fatty acids (or vitamin F). Skin that breaks out in blemishes may be desperate for more vitamin A, while a tendency to produce excessive oil is often tempered by a good dose of B vitamins. A sure way to improve the quality of your skin is to nourish it from both inside and out.

FRESH START

The kind of diet that builds beautiful skin enhances health at every level. While we need small quantities of every single essential nutrient, the skin relies on some of these for its wellbeing more than others. Certain foods are particularly rich in skin-nourishing nutrients so be sure to include them in your diet.

But before filling your shopping basket with skin superfoods, here are a few general guidelines for healthy eating.

Fresh is best ~ Fruits, vegetables and cereals are at their most nutritious when just picked or harvested. Nutrients are lost during storage and the longer foods stay on the shelf, the more depleted they become. For optimal freshness choose fruits and vegetables as they come into season and whenever possible pick your own.

Opt for organic ~ Pesticides and preservatives may yield better looking, longer lasting foods but to the body these chemicals are alien and seen as toxins. Their presence may upset the healthy functioning of tissues, and that includes skin. More alarmingly, some pesticides such as lindane are known carcinogens and can increase the risk of cancer. Whenever possible choose organically grown produce. Even small changes make a big difference.

Close to nature ~ Choose foods that are whole and unadulterated, as nature intended. Processing frequently destroys nutrients. When flour is refined and bleached it loses 70–90 per

— Blueprint for healthy eating —

- Fresh fruits and vegetables in rainbow colours of green, red, orange, yellow, purple and blue. Go for five portions a day or more.

- Nuts and seeds including almonds, walnuts, pistachios, pecans, hazelnuts, brazil nuts and pumpkin, sesame and sunflower seeds. Eat daily as snacks or sprinkle over cereals and into salads.

- Wholegrain cereals and breads such as oats, rye, wheat, barley, brown rice and buckwheat. Eat daily for constant energy.

- Pulses, legumes and beans. Eat daily; they combine well with vegetables.

- Fish including oily varieties such as salmon, sardines, mackerel, and shellfish such as prawns, scallops and mussels. Eat three times a week, ideally.

- Organic and free-range eggs. Eat up to four times a week.

- Organic and free-range poultry, duck and game birds. Eat up to three times a week.

- Organic red meat such as lamb, beef and pork. Ideally eat once or twice a week.

- Dairy products including natural live yoghurt, organic milk, low-fat cheese and unsalted butter. Live yoghurt can be eaten daily, but other dairy products should be eaten sparingly.

cent of its original B complex vitamins and many minerals. In the raw, sugar cane contains calcium, iron, potassium and sulphur, nutrients the body needs to metabolise this sweet stuff. When purified, these essential nutrients are washed away. Our biochemistry is attuned to foods as they occur in nature. Vitality comes naturally when we give our body what it really needs.

Cook it yourself ~ Time is precious and ready-made meals are a tempting alternative to home cooking. But commercially prepared dishes can be spiced up with artificial colourings, flavourings and preservatives that may trigger sensitivity and skin reactions. Simple dishes prepared from fresh ingredients like salads and stir-fries can be knocked up in minutes and are infinitely more nourishing.

Essential Skin Nutrients

AMINO ACIDS

Skin-perfecting qualities ~ Amino acids are the building blocks of enzymes and the internal cell structures. Strong, healthy skin relies on a good supply of these nutrients.

Time to top up ~ When skin is dull and lacks vitality.

Best natural sources ~ There are eight essential amino acids that we must get from our diet, and a further 12 that our bodies can make. Fish, meat, eggs and dairy products provide all the essential ones, while beans, pulses and vegetables need to be eaten in combination to get the full spectrum.

VITAMINS

Vitamin A/Beta-carotene

Skin-perfecting qualities ~ A potent antioxidant and anti-ageing nutrient which helps preserve skin's youthful looks.

Vitamin A can be made from beta-carotene which is found in any green, yellow and orange fruits and vegetables. Excessive amounts of pure vitamin A can overload tissues and cause toxicity, so increasing beta-carotene intake is a much safer way of keeping levels at an optimum.

This nutrient plays an essential role in keeping skin healthy and well-protected. It ensures the cells rising to the surface remain supple so the skin feels soft and smooth. Beta-carotene provides an element of sun protection and protects against sun damage.

On the surface ~ Retinoic acid, a vitamin A derivative, used to treat acne and reverse some of the age-accelerating damage inflicted by the sun. Chemical cousins such as retinol have similar but milder properties.

Time to top up ~ If skin is dry, rough and breaks out in spots. When in short supply, cells become hard and flaky before they reach the surface. They block the pores which encourages spots and prevents the oils from flowing freely. It's also important to top up when your skin is exposed to strong sun.

Best natural sources ~ See chart on page 56.

B complex vitamins

Skin-perfecting qualities ~ B vitamins help rebuild and repair skin tissue. They also generate the energy needed to keep cells working, keep nerves healthy and help oxygenate the skin. The term encompasses the family of B vitamins which include thiamin (B1), riboflavin (B2), niacin (B3), pantothenic acid (B5), pyriodoxine (B6), cyanocobalamin (B12), choline and folic acid.

On the surface ~ Panthenol, a relation of vitamin B5, is used in skin creams for its softening and fortifying properties.

Time to top up ~ If skin is flushed red or pale, greasy (especially at the sides of the nose), scaly and flaky. Lack of B vitamins can cause dry and cracking lips. Stress, alcohol and the contraceptive pill increase the need for B vitamins.

Best natural sources ~ See chart on page 56.

Vitamin C

Skin-perfecting qualities ~ A powerful antioxidant nutrient and cleanser. Vitamin C is used by the fibroblasts in the dermis to make collagen, which keeps the skin strong and springy. It also protects from stress, reduces allergic reactions by neutralising the arch-irritant histamine and helps flush toxins from the tissues.

On the surface ~ Vitamin C can be taken up by the skin and then moves into general circulation. It strengthens small capillaries, reinforces collagen, reduces inflammation and reverses sun damage. Vitamin C is used in moisturisers and nourishing creams.

Time to top up ~ If skin bruises easily, wounds heal slowly and wrinkles are beginning to appear. Stress, infections, pollution and sun exposure increase the need for this nutrient.

Best natural sources ~ See chart on page 56.

Vitamin E

Skin-perfecting qualities ~ A super antioxidant which protects the cell membranes from damage. Vitamin E can prolong cell life, promote healing and reduce scarring. It helps to rebalance and improve a variety of skin conditions including acne, eczema and psoriasis. A valuable treatment for sunburn.

On the surface ~ Applying oils rich in vitamin E to the skin promotes softness, retards ageing and supports healing.

Time to top up ~ When skin is too oily or too dry, bruises easily and suffers from poor circulation. Also top up when your skin is exposed to the sun.

Best natural sources ~ See chart on page 56.

ESSENTIAL FATTY ACIDS (vitamin F)

Skin-perfecting qualities ~ These nutrients are used to build cell membranes. Two essential fatty acids – linoleic acid and alpha-linolenic acid – must be obtained from the diet. In the body they are made into other health-enhancing substances.

Linoleic acid (an omega 6 fatty acid) is turned into gamma-linolenic acid (GLA), also found in evening primrose and borage oils. Alpha-linolenic acid (an omega 3 fatty acid) is turned into eicosapentanoeic acid (EPA) and docosa-hexaenoic acid (DHA), also found in oily, cold-water fish. The omega 6 and 3 fatty acids work together to keep the skin soft, velvety and resistant to the dehydrating effects of the elements.

Hormone-like chemicals called prosta-glandins are also made from the essential fatty acids. These support the immune system, enhance energy production, influence fluid balance and control inflammation.

On the surface ~ Omega 6 fatty acids help to strengthen, soften and moisturise when applied to the skin and are used in nourishing creams and moisturisers, but omega 3 fatty acids work best from within.

Time to top up ~ When skin is dehydrated rough, inflamed and prone to sensitivity reactions. Eczema often flares up when these nutrients are in short supply.

Best natural sources ~ See chart on page 56.

MINERALS

Calcium

Skin-perfecting qualities ~ Works closely alongside vitamin C to make collagen and other nutrients to keep the skin healthy. Keeps the blood capillaries in good condition and is involved in skin healing.

Time to top up ~ When skin is stressed and needs calming.

Best natural sources ~ See chart on page 56.

Iron

Skin-perfecting qualities ~ The key mineral in the pigment that carries oxygen in the blood to the skin. Lack of iron results in weakness, fatigue and poor resistance to infection. Iron ensures skin glows from within.

Time to top up ~ When skin is pale and lacks vitality and there are dark rings under the eyes.

Best natural sources ~ See chart on page 56.

Magnesium

Skin-perfecting qualities ~ Involved in repairing and maintaining skin cells, magnesium helps to balance hormones and buffers the effects of stress. Works alongside calcium, the B vitamins and essential fatty acids to keep skin healthy.

Time to top up ~ When skin is stressed and suffering from pre-menstrual upheavals such as puffiness and pimples.

Best natural sources ~ See chart on page 56.

Selenium

Skin-perfecting qualities ~ Forms part of an important antioxidant enzyme called glutathione peroxidase which protects skin from damage that accelerates ageing and wrinkle formation. Helps to preserve skin's youthful appearance.

Time to top up ~ When skin is dry and flaky and during sun exposure. Also when skin heals slowly and is susceptible to infection.

Best natural sources ~ See chart on page 56.

Silica

Skin-perfecting qualities ~ A constituent of sand and rocks that is found in tiny amounts as silica (silicon dioxide) in every tissue, especially the skin, and is essential for cell growth. Silica helps to keep skin smooth and supple.

Time to top up ~ When skin is susceptible to allergic rashes.

Best natural sources ~ See chart on page 56.

Sulphur

Skin-perfecting qualities ~ Renowned beauty mineral needed for making collagen and important anti-ageing antioxidant enzymes. Helps to rid the body of toxins. Spa waters rich in sulphur are thought to benefit skin conditions such as psoriasis, eczema and dermatitis. In creams, sulphur enhances moisturising power and may help to prevent allergies and treat burns.

Time to top up ~ When skin is dry, rough and inclined to be sensitive.

Best natural sources ~ See chart on page 56.

Zinc

Skin-perfecting qualities ~ Vital for growth and repair of skin. Plays an essential role in healing. Prevents stretch marks and scar-tissue formation. Zinc supports the immune system to resist infections.

Time to top up ~ When skin is excessively dry or oily, heals slowly and is prone to infections.

Best natural sources ~ See chart on page 56.

SKIN NUTRIENTS

SKIN VITAMINS	BEST NATURAL FOOD SOURCES
Vitamin A	eggs, butter, cream, full-fat milk, liver, kidney, herring, mackerel
Beta-carotene	carrots, spinach, cabbage, sweet potatoes, pumpkin, mangoes, apricots, cantaloupe melon
B complex vitamins	wholegrain cereals, brown rice, peas, beans, lentils, green leafy vegetables, meat, eggs, bananas, avocado, nuts, seeds
Vitamin C	lemons, grapefruit, oranges, mandarins, limes, kiwi fruits, rosehips, Brussels sprouts, peppers, watercress, spinach, potatoes, tomatoes
Vitamin E	cold-pressed vegetable oils (especially almond), wheatgerm, brown rice, egg yolks, asparagus
Essential fatty acids	sunflower and pumpkin seeds, linseeds (flax), hemp oil, nuts (especially walnuts), soya beans, leafy vegetables, oily fish
Calcium	cheese, milk, fresh fish, chickpeas, pulses, figs, leafy and root vegetables, oatmeal, sesame seeds
Iron	lamb's liver, sardines, shellfish, wholegrains, cocoa solids, raisins and sultanas, parsley, beetroot, broccoli, cabbage
Magnesium	almonds, soya beans, wholegrains, green leafy vegetables, shrimps
Selenium	fish, shellfish, wholegrains, eggs, milk, fruits, vegetables
Silica	oats, barley, millet, wholewheat, onions, beetroot, horsetail herb
Sulphur	pure spring water, eggs, meat, onions, alfalfa, cabbage, broccoli, watercress
Zinc	fresh oysters, shrimps, ginger root, lamb, beef, chicken, pecans, split peas, brazil nuts, almonds, walnuts, hazelnuts, buckwheat, wholewheat, corn, green peas, turnips, potatoes, garlic, carrots, sea vegetables

Super Skin Foods

WHAT ARE PHYTONUTRIENTS?

For years researchers have noticed that some fruits and vegetables have exceptional health-enhancing and therapeutic properties which cannot be attributed to their vitamins and minerals alone.

New research reveals that these superfoods contain special biologically active substances known as phytochemicals or phytonutrients. In plants these chemicals offer protection from things that jeopardise the plant's survival such as environmental pollutants, strong sunlight, bacteria and viruses.

These phytochemicals are proving to be the most promising tools we possess when it comes to preserving and enhancing our sense of well-being. The following plant foods have amazing powers for perfecting skin, so tap into nature's bounty.

Algae

At first glance the green slimy stuff that flourishes in lakes holds little promise as a superfood, but looks are deceptive. Two particular algae have been prized for centuries as superfoods and are now recognised as being rich sources of essential skin nutrients. They should be available at your local healthfood store or you can order direct from stockists (see pages 197–9).

Spirulina, a blue-green algae, is rich in essential amino acids, beta-carotene, chlorophyll, gamma-linolenic acid (GLA), trace minerals and enzymes. It also provides vitamins B1, B2, B6, D, E and K, and is the richest plant source of vitamin B12.

Spirulina helps cells regenerate, reverses deterioration associated with ageing, strengthens the immune system and helps digestion. Buy only the purest organically grown spirulina bearing the Soil Association's seal of approval. Hawaiian pacifica spirulina has been approved for purity.

Chlorella, a green algae, boasts such a complete spectrum of nutrients that it has been researched as a potential space food. Like spirulina it is rich in essential amino acids, vitamins, minerals and chlorophyll. In addition chlorella contains a growth factor (CGF) which appears to aid the uptake of nucleic acids, the building blocks of DNA and RNA (the cell's genetic material). This makes it helpful for repairing the kind of cell damage associated with ageing.

Almonds

Highly valued in traditional Indian medicine (Ayurveda), almonds are one of the few alkaline nuts. They are a particularly good source of magnesium, a skin nutrient which is often referred to as nature's tranquilliser because of its calming influence on the nerves. Almonds are rich in vitamin E and contain valuable quantities of calcium, zinc, potassium, folic acid, vitamins B2 and B3. In skin treatments, ground almonds and almond oil have softening and nourishing qualities.

Apples and pears

These orchard fruits are both good sources of beta-carotene, vitamin C, B1, magnesium, potassium, calcium and folic acid. Pears are also high in iodine which helps to regulate energy levels. Their skins contain pectin, a soluble fibre which absorbs toxins and speeds their removal from the intestinal tract. The slightly sour-tasting malic and tartaric acid in apples prevents fermentation and bacterial proliferation in the gut, which in turn keeps the digestive system healthy. While apple juice cleanses the liver, the juice of pears is

said to be helpful for relieving eczema. Applied to the skin they are moisturising and nourishing.

Avocado

Avocados are particularly rich in vitamins A, B, C and E, along with potassium, plus smaller quantities of iron and vitamin K. They have a balanced acid/alkaline content and produce an oil that is renowned for its skin-beautifying properties. Mashed to a pulp, avocado flesh makes a nourishing treat for dry, lack-lustre skin.

Carrots

Carrots owe their brilliant orange colour to beta-carotene, the precursor of vitamin A. They also contain alpha-carotene another carotenoid with cancer-preventing properties. Together these phytonutrients can boost the skin's natural sun protection factor (SPF) and reduce sun damage. Carrots are rich in vitamins B1, B2 and the minerals potassium, sodium and silicon.

Regularly nibbling carrots or drinking carrot juice improves skin's appearance and helps clear spots and blemishes.

Applying carrot oil to the skin helps smooth out wrinkles and brighten a sallow complexion.

Cherries

Cherries are renowned for their skin-beautifying

qualities. As well as being rich in antioxidant vitamins A and C, cherries supply useful quantities of B vitamins plus the minerals calcium, magnesium, potassium and iron. Cherries also support the cleansing activities of the liver, kidneys and intestines.

On the outside, mashed cherries will brighten and refine a dull, sallow skin.

Lemons and limes

These citrus fruits have many skin-beautifying qualities. Both are rich sources of vitamin C which keeps collagen in good condition.

Lemons also contain small amounts of calcium and potassium. Lemon juice is slightly antiseptic. It helps cleanse the blood and liver, making it an asset to any detox regime. Sipping lemon juice in hot water first thing each morning helps preserve inner purity. The pith is rich in bioflavonoids, phytonutrients that strengthen tiny blood capillaries and prevent unattractive broken veins. Swept over the skin, lemon juice restores the acid mantle, refines the pores and prevents pimples. Used regularly it evens irregular pigmentation and is said to smooth out wrinkles.

Lime blossom or linden makes wonderfully soothing infusions which relieve stress and promote sleep. On the skin this floral infusion

softens, lubricates and is believed to encourage cell regeneration. It also helps relieve the symptoms of eczema.

Oats

Oats are one of nature's most nutritious cereals. They are rich in slow-release carbohydrates so supply a steady stream of glucose to the blood over a relatively long period which gives long-lasting energy. They are also packed with energy-generating and nerve-fortifying B vitamins, as well as the minerals calcium, magnesium, iron, manganese and silica. Together they strengthen the skin from within.

Although high in fibre, oats also soothe the digestive system. And Tincture of Oats (*Avena Sativa*) is a helpful, calming and reviving remedy recommended for nervous exhaustion.

On the skin, oats have soothing and moisturising properties. Oatmeal makes a soft skin scrub. When wrapped in muslin to hang in the bath, it makes a soothing soak for eczema.

Sea vegetables

Marine plants gather and concentrate minerals in the sea, presenting them in a form that the body finds easy to assimilate.

Seaweed synthesises B complex vitamins including vitamin B12 (missing from land vegetables), plus vitamins A, C, D, E and K, as well as substantial quantities of protein. It is particularly rich in iodine, a mineral needed by the thyroid gland for regulating metabolism. A gelatinous substance called alginic acid is a power cleanser as it absorbs toxins and speeds their removal from the body.

The best edible varieties are:

Nori, a Japanese seaweed available in wafer-thin sheets;

Laver, traditionally fried with oats to make laverbread;

Dulse, deep red in colour and slightly spicy;

Samphire, grows along the seashore and makes a delicious vegetable dish.

Seaweed face and body masks have highly nourishing and deep-cleansing properties (see page 44).

Strawberries

These summer fruits are exceptionally rich in vitamin C as well as silicon, a mineral useful for repairing and strengthening connective tissue. For this reason they work wonders for keeping wrinkles at bay.

Strawberries are also rich in potassium, vitamin B3, folic acid and beta-carotene. Like other blue-, purple- and red-berry fruits they are rich in phytonutrients called anthocyanidins. These are powerful antioxidants that offer protection from sun damage, prevent inflammation, strengthen blood capillaries and may even reverse some aspects of ageing. They also have valuable cleansing qualities.

Applied to the skin strawberries cleanse, refine and restore brightness.

Super seeds

Plant seeds are nutritional treasure troves and their oils have superb skin-conditioning qualities.

Sunflower seeds are rich in protein, vitamins A, D, E, several B vitamins, calcium, magnesium, iron and zinc, all essential skin nutrients. They are also an exceptionally rich source of omega 6 linoleic acid.

Sunflower seed oil is light and sinks into the skin easily, making it ideal for moisturisers and creams.

Flax seeds (linseeds) were being cultivated over 2,000 years ago and were once a valued part of our diet. Research reveals them to be the richest natural source of skin-softening omega 3 alpha-linolenic acid.

These tiny golden seeds boast a full complement of essential amino acids. They are rich in vitamin E and B vitamins, calcium, magnesium and sulphur. They contain a soluble fibre called mucilage which soothes the digestive tract.

Flax seeds are also the most abundant source of lignans, phyto-oestrogens which help to keep the skin soft and youthful. They are currently being investigated for their ability to prevent hormone-related cancers.

Hemp seeds are close cousins of flax seeds and contain omega 3 and 6 fatty acids in a ratio of 3:1, making it the perfect skin drink. Hemp oil, as its colour suggests, is high in chlorophyll and appears to be helpful for preventing and alleviating eczema.

Tomatoes

These sun-ripened fruits have long been regarded as an anti-wrinkle treatment. Tomatoes are now known to be rich in the phytonutrient lycopene, a powerful antioxidant carotenoid which prevents free-radical damage and undoes sun damage.

Other noteworthy nutrients are vitamin C, calcium and potassium.

Tomatoes are natural cleansers with antiseptic and alkaline properties which help to purify the blood and encourage detoxification. They also protect and strengthen the digestive tract.

As tomatoes interfere with calcium absorption, do not eat more than four a day.

Watercress

This plant is brimming with the super-cleansing pigment chlorophyll, plus other skin vitamins and minerals. Watercress is especially rich in beta-carotene, vitamin C, zinc, iron, potassium and iodine.

It contains a potent phytonutrient called phenethyl isothiocyanate which neutralises the dangerous carcinogens in tobacco.

Watercress compresses help to heal acne and other skin conditions.

Wheatgrass

Lush young shoots of sprouting wheat yield a vivid green juice brimming with chlorophyll and a full spectrum of essential skin nutrients from beta-carotene and vitamin C through to vitamins B and E, plus 90 different minerals including calcium, magnesium, potassium and iron. It is rich in active enzymes which aid digestion.

A potent cleanser with antiseptic properties, wheatgrass purifies the blood, unearths deep-seated toxins and cleans up after bacterial and viral infections.

From the inside and out, wheatgrass clarifies the skin and is helpful for treating acne. Try pouring the juice over you in a tub of warm water. Soak in it for 15–20 minutes and rinse off with a cold shower.

Skin Drinks

Freshly squeezed fruit and vegetable juices are pure liquid nutrition.

They contain concentrated amounts of vitamins, minerals and health-promoting phytonutrients such as chlorophyll, carotenoids and bioflavonoids in a pure water suspension.

Drunk on a regular basis they will help to cleanse and nourish the skin from within. They have remarkable powers for revitalising complexions that have lost their natural radiance through stress, overwork or illness.

CONCENTRATED GOODNESS

Most naturopaths (practitioners who use the healing powers of nature) believe that nutrients occurring naturally in foods are bound up in complexes which the body recognises and readily absorbs. Vitamins and minerals in supplements, on the other hand, are often synthesised and mixed with fillers which the digestive system may reject. At times when your body needs an extra nutritional boost, it may be better to drink a glass or two of fresh juice than swallow a couple of pills. Naturally occurring nutrients tend to be present in a balanced form

that is in tune with the body's own needs. Raw-food enthusiasts also maintain that fresh fruits and vegetables possess a life force that helps to revive and rekindle our own energy levels.

People who drink fresh juices on a daily basis tend to have clear, radiant skin and boundless vitality.

SMOOTH OPERATORS

Mixing milk or natural yoghurt with fresh fruits and juices creates deliciously creamy blends which are both filling and highly nutritious. Smoothies are essentially exotic milkshakes and have always been popular in the Caribbean where they are often made with fresh coconut milk. They make an ideal breakfast or snack when the weather is hot or when you are too busy to prepare a proper meal.

If you are prone to catarrh and sinus congestion, naturopaths advise avoiding cow's milk as it tends to be mucus forming. Soya, rice and almond milk are ideal alternatives and taste just as good when whizzed up with fresh fruit.

Juicing tips

SPRING TONICS	SUMMER COOLERS	AUTUMN ENERGISERS	WINTER WARMERS
Blend:	**Blend:**	**Blend:**	**Blend:**
145ml (5fl oz) carrot juice	175ml (6fl oz) tomato juice	175ml (6fl oz) carrot juice	115ml (4fl oz) carrot juice
50ml (2fl oz) celery juice	25ml (1fl oz) spinach juice	50ml (2fl oz) beetroot juice	50ml (2fl oz) red pepper juice
25ml (1fl oz) watercress juice	25ml (1fl oz) watercress juice		25ml (1fl oz) watercress or parsley juice
			1 clove garlic
Blend:	**Blend:**	**Blend:**	**Blend:**
115ml (4fl oz) grapefruit juice	115ml (4fl oz) milk or natural yoghurt	175ml (6fl oz) apple juice	1 banana
80ml (3fl oz) mandarin or orange juice	50ml (2fl oz) mango juice	50ml (2fl oz) blackcurrant or blackberry juice	115ml (4fl oz) pineapple juice
25ml (1fl oz) lime juice	50ml (2fl oz) raspberry juice		50ml (2fl oz) mango juice

§ Choose the freshest fruits and vegetables as they will be richer in essential nutrients. Vitamin C especially deteriorates a little every day the produce is kept. Make exactly the right amount of juice and drink straight away – do not save it for later.

§ Use organic produce whenever possible. Juicing will concentrate any pesticide residues along with nutrients. Alternatively remove the peel and/or soak in pesticide-removing 'Vegewash' (see pages 197–9 for stockist information).

§ Make sure fruit is really ripe and succulent for juicing.

§ When juicing citrus fruits, be sure to add in the pith as it is rich in capillary-strengthening bioflavonoids. Use the whole fruit whenever possible as many nutrients are present within or lie just beneath the skin.

§ Avoid mixing fruit and vegetable juices as in combination these tend to cause flatulence. The exception is apple and carrot which harmonise perfectly.

§ Aim to drink equal amounts of both fruit and vegetable juices rather than just one variety to get a good spread of nutrients. Remember fruits also tend to be high in natural sugars.

Strike a Balance

In the West, a balanced diet is one that supplies all the nutrients we
need to stay healthy. But in Eastern countries the interpretation of
balance is quite different.

In Traditional Chinese Medicine foods are classified in terms of their influence on the body's energies or chi. The right combination of foods preserves a sense of wellbeing by keeping the chi energy in balance.

According to Chinese medical thinking, the body's life force or chi energy flows along channels called meridians. When the energy becomes blocked or stagnates, it gives rise to various emotional and health problems which are reflected in the skin. For instance, from the Chinese medical viewpoint spots and skin blemishes may be due to an energy blockage in the liver and gall bladder meridian. A corrective diet uses foods that restore the flow of energy in this particular meridian and so clear the complexion.

It is a good idea to eat a spectrum of coloured foods relating to the five Chinese elements as they will help to balance the key meridians.

COLOURFUL FOODS FOR BALANCE AND HEALTH

Element/Colour	Foods	Meridian
Fire/red	tomatoes, red peppers	balances heart and small intestine
Earth/yellow, orange	sweet potato, sweetcorn, orange and yellow peppers, pumpkin, squash, tangerines	balances spleen and stomach
Metal/white	water chestnuts, asparagus, button mushrooms, milk	balances lungs and large intestine
Wood/green	chives, chicory, celery, spinach, kale	balances liver and gall bladder
Water/blue, black	clams, mussels, black sesame seeds, black beans, chestnuts, black grapes, plums, blueberries	balances kidneys and bladder

FLAVOURFUL FOODS FOR BALANCE AND HEALTH

FLAVOUR	FOODS	MERIDIAN
Bitter	lettuce, radish leaves, vinegar	balances heart and small intestine
Sweet	honey, cherries, melon, banana	balances spleen and stomach
Pungent	chives, cloves, parsley, coriander, mint	balances lungs and large intestine
Sour	lemon, pear, plum	balances liver and gall bladder
Salty	salt, kelp, seaweed	balances kidneys and bladder

OPPOSITES ATTRACT

In Chinese philosophy everything in life including ourselves and the food we eat is described in terms of two opposing principles – Yin and Yang. Yin = female, dark, cold, negative, passive, earth; Yang = male, light, hot, strong, positive, active, sun.

Keeping these two energy forces in balance is thought to hold the key to inner harmony and a sense of all-pervading equilibrium. Skin that is flushed and high-coloured suggests an excess of Yang energy which can be countered by emphasising cooling Yin foods. On the other hand, when skin is pale and washed out it may benefit from a zing of fiery Yang energy.

Similarly, eating a diet composed predominantly of Yin or Yang foods may provoke an existing skin problem. As most Westerners are unfamiliar with the energy qualities of different foods the safest way to strike a balance is to have lots of variety in your diet. Try to strike balance between eating hot, spicy 'Yang' foods like garlic and ginger, and cool, watery 'Yin' foods like cucumber and watermelon.

FULL OF FLAVOUR

A well-balanced diet is rich in flavour, too. Variety not only satisfies all the taste buds; in Chinese philosophy different flavours also hone in on the various meridians and help to rebalance their chi energy. During the day aim to eat foods of all flavours to preserve a sense of balance.

The Perfect pH

Just as our skin has an optimum pH value so does our blood.

This was the view of Dr William Hay, one of the pioneers of food combining. Whereas our skin is naturally mildly acidic, Hay proposed that good health goes hand in hand with blood that has a mildly alkaline pH of around 7.5.

If blood pH drops below 7 and becomes slightly acidic we are more likely to feel tired, irritable and susceptible to health problems.

Many factors including stress and the kind of foods we eat can affect the blood pH value. Hay suggested that the diet most conducive to natural vitality and radiant skin is composed of alkaline- and acid-forming foods in a ratio of 4:1.

ACID- AND ALKALINE-FORMING FOODS

Acid	Neutral	Alkaline
cheese	oils	vegetables (especially carrots,
eggs	butter	potatoes, avocados,
fish	tea	spinach and beetroot
shellfish	coffee	fruits (except plums and
meat		cranberries)
poultry		pulses – lentils, beans (except
grains		broad and butter beans)
olives		nuts (except hazelnuts
		and walnuts)

Seasonal supplements

Seasonal weather changes can stress the skin but adjusting your diet throughout the year helps it to cope from within.

Drying winter conditions call for a dietary boost of essential fatty acids and beta-carotene or vitamin A to help keep the skin soft and supple. At this time of year eat plenty of seeds, nuts, oily fish, orange fruits and vegetables.

In the summer months when the UV rays are strongest and at their most damaging, skin will benefit from extra antioxidant nutrients which protect against sun damage (see page 131). Seek out foods rich in vitamins A, C, E, selenium and protective plant carotenoids in tomatoes, spinach, kale, pumpkin, carrots, broccoli, sweet potato and cantaloupe melon.

Take two tablespoons of flax oil every day during the winter months. Use it in salad dressings and pour over steamed vegetables. Never cook with this oil as heating destroys its essential nutrients.

Eat fruits and vegetables that are in season. This has two important benefits. Firstly, the fresher they are the more nutrients they contain.

The longer the time spent in transit and storage, the higher the loss of certain nutrients particularly vitamin C and certain B vitamins. Secondly, nature also has a habit of providing us with what our bodies need at the right time. Root vegetables in the autumn and winter are rich in energy-sustaining carbohydrates, summer fruits bursting with moisture, vitamin C and antioxidants are just what's needed in the hotter months.

Go with the flow. In Chinese and Indian medicine the kind of diet that preserves balance changes throughout the year. What you eat should therefore reflect the seasons. In winter, Yin energy predominates. This is a time for eating warm, cooked foods like stews, casseroles and bakes prepared from beef, lamb and root vegetables. In summer, Yang energy predomi-nates. This is a time for eating cooling, uncooked foods such as raw vegetable salads and succulent fruits like watermelon.

In spring and autumn go for a combination of Yin and Yang foods. Try lightly cooked dishes of chicken with seasonal vegetables and eat plenty of fresh fruit – cherries, grapes, peaches, pineapples and plums.

These are general guidelines for maintaining a sense of wellbeing and keeping the skin looking its best. A Chinese herbal practitioner will go into much greater depth when looking for the source of imbalance that gives rise to a particular skin problem. In addition to making dietary recommendations, he or she may prescribe various herbal remedies designed to bring the energies back into balance. For information on finding a practitioner, see page 199.

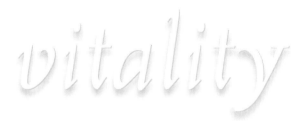

Having It All

A diet rich in nutrient-packed foods is the first step towards nourishing your skin. Good digestion is the second for it ensures these nutrients actually reach their destination.

When foods are eaten and pass into the digestive system they are mixed with a variety of different digestive enzymes. These enzymes break down the various food components and release nutrients so they can be taken up through the gut wall and pass into the bloodstream. Following absorption, nutrients are carried to where they are most needed. But the course of digestion does not always run smoothly. Bloating, indigestion and feeling heavy after a meal are tell-tale signs that something is amiss.

These problems are so common that we often regard them as normal, but this is not so. As well as feeling satisfied we should also feel light and energised after a meal.

Ways to improve digestion

- ♦ Chew every mouthful – digestion begins in the mouth. Chewing breaks down food and mixes it with saliva which contains a carbohydrate-digesting enzyme called ptyalin.

- ♦ Don't eat in a hurry. Stress inhibits the proper flow of digestive enzymes which is why we get a dry mouth when anxious or fearful. If there isn't enough time to relax, sit down and enjoy a meal in peace, opt for light snacks until the moment presents itself.

- ♦ Eat little and often. Eating large quantities at one meal can place a tremendous strain on your body's digestive capacity. Grazing encourages better nutrient assimilation.

- ♦ Include raw food in your diet. The cells of fresh fruits and vegetables are rich in live active enzymes which are released during chewing. These enzymes have the power to break down proteins, carbohydrates and fats so they effectively enhance our own digestive powers. Amazingly these enzymes appear to pass unharmed into the small intestine where they help to create conditions favourable to good digestion.

  Cooking destroys these enzymes. Sprouting grains and seeds on the other hand turn them into powerhouses of active digestion-aiding enzymes.

Keep it simple. According to the principles of food combining, eating foods rich in protein and carbohydrate together interferes with the proper digestion of both. As a general rule it helps to keep your meal uncomplicated, i.e. don't make elaborate dishes with lots of different ingredients. Simply prepared fish cooked with herbs or pasta with tomato sauce, for example, will be much easier to digest. Eat fruits separately or at least an hour after a main meal.

Replenish the good bugs. There are millions of bacteria in the digestive tract which play a positive role in defending you from unfriendly microbes, digesting fibre and making small quantities of vitamin B12. These good bacteria belong to the *Lactobaccillus* and *Bifidus* families. Gastric upsets such as holiday diarrhoea can wipe out vast quantities of good bacteria. When this happens we tend to suffer from wind and gastric discomfort. From time to time it helps to replenish the good bugs. Eat live natural yoghurt each morning and consider taking a short course of probiotics – three capsules a day for two weeks.

Natural digestive aids

Eat a few slices of fresh pineapple or papaya after a meal. These fruits are rich in protein-digesting enzymes called bromelain and papain respectively. In traditional cuisine they are often used to tenderise meats and will aid the digestion of protein-rich foods.

Flavour your food with herbs and spices. While their delicious aromas get the saliva flowing before a meal, certain active chemicals aid the digestive process. Fennel, ginger and cayenne pepper are particularly known for their digestion-enhancing qualities.

If you are prone to indigestion introduce partially fermented foods such as yoghurt, cottage cheese, miso, tofu and soya sauce to your diet. Already semi-digested, they place less stress on your own digestive enzymes and readily relinquish their nutrients.

– Tip –

To aid digestion, try sipping peppermint tea after a meal or make an infusion of freshly grated ginger and sweeten with honey to taste.

Skin Nourishing Treatments

Some nutrients do sink into the skin and help to nourish the cells. The best time to use skin-nourishing preparations is just before going to bed so they can assist with the cell regeneration that takes place as you sleep.

— Recipes —

NOURISHING SERUM

1 tablespoon aloe vera gel
2 tablespoons rosehip infusion
10 drops carrot oil
1 capsule vitamin E oil
10 drops evening primrose oil
4 drops rose essential oil
2 drops ylang ylang essential oil

Spoon the aloe vera gel into a small glass bowl and stir in 2 tablespoons of rosehip infusion. Now add in the carrot, vitamin E (pierce the capsule to squeeze out the oil) and evening primrose oil before finally scenting with rose and ylang ylang essential oils. If possible decant into a pump dispenser. Keep in the fridge and use within a month.

For a week, smooth a few drops over your face every night just before going to bed to revitalise your complexion or whenever your skin is looking tired and under-nourished.

SKIN SUPPLEMENT

1 tablespoon finely ground almonds
1 tablespoon live natural yoghurt
1 or 2 fresh strawberries, raspberries, blueberries or pitted cherries
10 drops carrot oil
4 drops rose essential oil

Place all the ingredients in a blender and whizz into a rich cream. Smear over your face. Place cottonwool pads soaked in rose water over your eyes and relax for 10–15 minutes to allow your skin to soak up the nutrients.

Rinse away with warm water and spray with the refresher of your choice (see pages 22–3). Use once a week for a nourishing boost.

vitality

radiant

CHAPTER FIVE

Oxygen

~

The Essence of Energy

Oxygen is the spark of life. Present in every breath we take, this ethereal element generates the energy that cells need to survive and thrive. Skin infused with energising oxygen exudes radiance and vitality. Air pollution, shallow breathing and inner tensions mean skin is often starved of this vital nutrient. Fresh air and exercise together with circulation-boosting herbs and essential oils can restore a healthy glow. An oxygen surge gives skin a new lease of life, so take a deep breath.

Be energised.

Essential O$_2$

We can live for several weeks without food, a day or two without
water, but only a few minutes without air.

Although it's invisible and untouchable, oxygen is all around us. The air we breathe is composed of around 21 per cent oxygen or O$_2$. The rest is made up of other gases, mostly nitrogen (78 per cent) together with small amounts of carbon dioxide (3 per cent) and traces of rarer elements such as helium and ozone.

Many ancient traditions taught that air, rather than food, gives us vitality. They showed great insight for oxygen is the vital spark that releases the energy necessary for powering all of life's processes.

In biochemical terms oxygen reacts with glucose to produce carbon dioxide, water and energy in the form of adenosine triphosphate (ATP). ATP is essentially a cell's energy currency. This process is going on constantly in every living cell of our bodies and to ensure it happens smoothly and swiftly we need a continuous supply of oxygen.

EVERY BREATH YOU TAKE

With every breath we draw oxygen deep down into the lungs. These organs, which look a little like spongy bunches of grapes, have very fine walls which are richly supplied with blood capillaries. Every minute the lungs receive as much blood as the rest of the entire body. Because the linings are so thin – just two cell layers thick – gases pass from the lungs to the bloodstream with ease. As oxygen moves into the blood, carbon dioxide, the by-product of energy production, diffuses out.

Oxygen is picked up by iron-rich haemoglobin, the ruby pigment present in red blood cells. It is then whisked swiftly away to every cell in the body in blood vessels that branch into smaller and smaller off-shoots before reaching the tiny capillaries just visible beneath the skin's surface. Here oxygen diffuses out of the blood and into the cells in exchange for carbon dioxide which is then carried back to the lungs. Then the whole process happens again.

SKIN LOVES FRESH AIR

In an ideal world the air would be as pure as nature intended. We feel energised simply being near the sea or in the mountains where the air is clear. Breaths of fresh air bring a blush of healthy colour to our cheeks and make our skin feel alive.

Nowadays, however, the air we breathe is often laden with stuff that shouldn't be there. Industry pours environmental pollutants into the atmosphere on a grand scale. Cars pump out fumes containing a cocktail of chemicals including carbon monoxide which actively competes with oxygen for haemoglobin. Other noxious chemicals include nitrogen oxide and hydrocarbons which irritate the lungs, trigger asthma attacks, exacerbate chest troubles and increase vulnerability to respiratory infections. In the presence of strong sunlight these chemicals react to make ozone which creates a hazy petrochemical smog that hangs in the air on hot summer days and causes breathing difficulties.

If you live in a traffic-congested city where air pollution is high, your skin and other tissues too may not receive their full quota of energising oxygen.

OPTIMISING OXYGEN

To ensure skin receives ample supplies of oxygen, it helps to keep the lungs in good condition. New research shows that eating fresh fruits and vegetables helps us to breathe more easily. The more you eat, the better your lung function will be. While vitamin A or beta-carotene keeps the linings of the lungs healthy and protects them from pollutant particles, other antioxidant nutrients such as vitamin C and E also appear to keep the airways healthy.

- Eat lots of fresh green vegetables, especially peas, broccoli, spring greens, dark green cabbage, parsley and courgettes.

- Drink plenty of tomato juice and use tomatoes in cooking.

- Nibble on sunflower seeds.

- Sip infusions of marshmallow or sip elderberry syrup diluted with pure spring water. Both marshmallow and elderberry are excellent tonics for the lungs.

The haemoglobin pigment in blood enables it to absorb four times as much oxygen as water. But haemoglobin relies on iron to do this and a lack of this mineral causes anaemia, the symptoms of which are similar to those of altitude sickness (oxygen levels at high altitudes are low). Lack of oxygen causes us to feel breathless, dizzy, lethargic, nauseous and faint on exertion. When skin does not get enough of this energising nutrient it becomes pale and lifeless. You can eat lots of iron-rich foods, but the mineral will not be properly absorbed unless vitamin C is present too.

– Purify the air –

§ Surround yourself with plants and flowers. While we take in oxygen (O_2) and breathe out carbon dioxide (CO_2) plants do it the other way around. They absorb our CO_2 and release pure O_2 back into the air. A NASA study has also found that house plants clear the air of indoor chemicals. Spider plants and peace lilies are particularly effective.

§ Detox your home. Indoor air can be ten times as polluted as that outdoors. Chemical pollutants come from household materials such as paints, plastics, varnishes and glues. We add to the load by spraying the air with aerosol cleaners, synthetic air-fresheners and other chemically laden household products.

§ Use pure and simple cleaning methods. Use a powerful vacuum cleaner to suck away the dust and dirt. Clean surfaces with a damp cloth soaked in water with a few drops of antiseptic lemon or lavender essential oil. Use good old-fashioned beeswax to buff up wooden furniture.

§ Avoid synthetic fragrances in soaps, perfume and other scented products. They are now so over-used that scientists can detect them in the air. Opt for pure plant essential oils to scent your skin and your home. They are better for you and the air we all breathe.

§ Give up smoking. Like car fumes, cigarette smoke contains carbon monoxide which deprives all the body's tissues of their rightful oxygen supply. Every inhalation also creates thousands of wrinkle-forming free radicals. No wonder smoking makes skin look dull and ten years older than its age.

Anaemia may also be due to a lack of vitamins B12 and folic acid. Vitamin B12 occurs naturally in animal foods such as meat, liver, dairy products and eggs. Spirulina and seaweed are the only plant exceptions. Lush leafy vegetables are an excellent source of iron, vitamin C and folic acid, so eat lots of spinach and greens to keep your skin well oxygenated.

76

Breathe Deeply

Full and rhythmical breathing works wonders for our skin.
It ensures the continuous flow of oxygen to cells and the swift removal
of carbon dioxide.

Breathing happens of its own accord but many things can upset normal breathing patterns without our even noticing. Step outdoors on a frosty day or into a very hot sauna and the temperature shock will automatically make you gasp and hold your breath. Laughing, speaking, singing and weeping all change our breathing, making inhalations deep and exhalations short and spasmodic.

When anxious, fearful, angry or frustrated, adrenaline starts to flow and our breaths become increasingly rapid and shallow. It's known as over-breathing or hyperventilation and makes the heart pound and head spin. This is what happens during a panic attack. Tribal shamans purposely breathe this way to alter states of consciousness. But fast and shallow breathing is bad news because it reduces the oxygen supply to all the tissues. When we live in a state of constant tension we fail to use our full breathing potential. The good news is that although breathing is automatic, we can consciously override it to make it better.

STRETCH AND GLOW

Yoga is possibly the oldest form of breathing therapy. This ancient system of exercise originates from India where it was developed and practised by yogis or spiritual men. They discovered how to energise and balance the mind, body and spirit through a combination of deep rhythmic breathing and certain stretching movements. The yogic term 'prana' is Sanskrit for breath yet it also refers to the life force or energy thought to pervade the universe. In Chinese philosophies this is known as chi or qi.

Yoga develops the art of slow deep 'ujjaya' breathing to stimulate the flow of prana around the body. This oxygenates the tissues and instils peace of mind. Meanwhile the postures literally squeeze tension out of the muscles and in doing so pave the way for freer, more relaxed day-to-day breathing.

The benefits reaped from practising yoga include smooth skin that exudes vitality, inner calm, greater energy and a lithe, supple body.

There are various different forms of yoga

varying from meditative (kripalu) to intensely aerobic (ashtanga). It is worth trying a few to find which one is best suited to you.

Ashtanga yoga ~ Also known as 'power yoga', it is vigorous and very demanding. You move fast and furiously from one pose to the next. Only for the very fit and supple.

Iyengar yoga ~ Precise poses that work wonders for improving posture and alignment. Controlled breathing is helpful for asthma. Highly therapeutic.

Kripalu yoga ~ Cultivates inner stillness and awareness of the breath or prana.

Sivananda yoga ~ Focuses on stretching and relaxation. Ideal for beginners as it revolves around twelve basic postures which include the headstand. When upside down the heart works as hard as if you were running. Chanting clears and quietens the mind.

Lazy yoga ~ Thai massage or Nuad Bo Rarn is an Eastern touch treatment, traditionally practised by Buddhist monks that is like having yoga done to you. It is similar to other oriental therapies because it works with the body's energies which are said to flow along 10 Sen lines (akin to meridians). Using firm but gentle pressure with hands, feet and elbows, the Thai masseur applies pressure to key points on the Sen lines and stretches your body into yoga positions, so squeezing away the tension and encouraging deeper breathing. It is a wonderfully energising treatment that restores the free flow of oxygen to the skin and other tissues.

Pilates ~ This is like a modern version of yoga. Movements are slow and controlled, each working in perfect unison with the in- and out-breath. Pilates centres the body, stretches every muscle, and works to create a body that is firm yet flexible. An excellent form of breathing therapy.

– How to enhance breathing –

- A normal breathing rate is 12–14 breaths a minute, so time yourself. If you breathe more frequently you need to slow down.

- When you inhale the ribs move up and out as the diaphragm contracts and becomes flatter. As you exhale the ribs move down and in as the diaphragm domes up as it relaxes. Breathing should be smooth and regular.

- To check your breathing lie on your back and place one hand flat on your tummy or upper abdomen and the other on your chest. As you breathe in your chest should barely move while your stomach rises. If it happens the other way round your breathing is shallow.

- As you breathe in try to visualise the air reaching deep into your lungs and allow your tummy to expand as fully as possible. As you breathe out imagine the stale air being squeezed from every nook and cranny while pulling your tummy flat. Pause for a second or two before breathing in again.

- Worry, internal struggles and deeply held tensions make the body more inflexible and interfere with our ability to breathe fully. Whenever you start to feel fraught, take a deep breath and as you exhale imagine blowing away the stress. Slow, regular breathing is one of the best forms of relaxation.

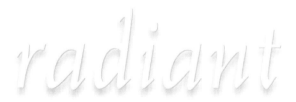

Exercise with Air

'Aerobic' literally means exercise with air.

This term has become synonymous with vigorous work-outs but aerobic exercise is essentially any movement-orientated exercise which makes the heart beat faster and the breathing rate increase. It is a wonderful way of getting blood and oxygen surging around the body.

When resting we breathe about 8 litres (14 pints) of air a minute but this can increase greatly during vigorous exercise. During exercise, blood flow to the skin increases primarily to cool the body. When this happens the skin cells enjoy a boost of energy and other essential nutrients. As we get fitter our breathing capacity and circulation increase. So, we take in more air and oxygen gets whisked to the skin more efficiently. Muscles become firmer and stronger giving skin better definition. If muscles shrink through inactivity, levels of sex hormones and steroid hormones also decrease proportionately. Many of these dwindling hormones play an important part in preserving water balance and youthful appearance of the skin.

The right moves

To reap these skin benefits exercise must become a part of your life, not something done on an occasional whim. Forget whatever happens to be in vogue.

- Discover an activity that you enjoy and fits in with your particular lifestyle, be it swimming, brisk walking, jogging, cycling, horse riding, skiing or working out in the gym.

- Try to exercise in the open air. In Chinese philosophy a lack of fresh air and exercise weakens the chi of breath. Indoor exercise may build fitness, but outdoor activities like cycling, walking and horse riding revitalise chi to energise mind and body.

- To cultivate and sustain fitness, aim for 20 minutes of aerobic exercise or an hour of brisk walking four times a week.

– Tip –

Bring colour to your complexion with an early morning face massage. Use a mixture of circling strokes, gentle squeezing, scissoring and pressure point stimulation.

Skin stimulation

Massage works wonders for oxygenating and energising the skin. It achieves this in two ways. Rubbing, kneading and light percussion movements stimulate the circulation and promote the flow of blood to the skin. Soothing strokes relax muscle tensions and free the breath.

Aim to massage your face for 5–10 minutes every day and bits of the body that are easy to reach. Work the following energising movements into your routine.

Circling strokes ~ Using the tips of fingers and palms of hands work over the skin using brisk circling movements. This instantly enhances skin tone.

Kneading ~ Squeeze skin between the thumb and fingers, then release as if you were kneading a piece of dough. Good for fleshy areas (hips, thighs, tummy, bottom) and for squeezing tension from the shoulders.

Percussion ~ Light 'hacking' movements using the sides of the hands are highly stimulating and invigorating. The wrists should be loose and flexible, the hands bouncy. Only use on fleshy areas.

— Recipe —

ROSY GLOW FACE OIL

2 drops lemon essential oil
4 drops rose essential oil
2 drops lavender essential oil
30ml (2 tablespoons) sweet almond oil
1 teaspoon jojoba oil

Blend the essential oils with the almond and jojoba oils. Massage into the face for 5 minutes, tissue off and then spray with floral water.

Pressure points ~ Both acupressure and shiatsu-style massage apply pressure to key points on the meridians to stimulate energy flow. To tone the lung meridian, work on an easily accessible point called Lung 7. With palms facing up, feel for the outer wrist bone (on thumb side) and apply firm and continuous finger or thumb pressure to it for about a minute.

Scissoring ~ A good movement for face massage. Interlock your first and second fingers from both hands and lay them flat against your forehead, then scissor briskly.

Energising Plants and Herbs

Various plant foods and herbs have a revitalising influence on the
blood and circulatory system and act as tonics.

Include these in your diet, especially during the cold winter months when blood flow is always more sluggish. Use these herbs when you need to restore skin's tone and vitality.

Beetroot ~ Rich in iron, vitamin C and folic acid. A good blood builder. Add beetroot juice to fresh vegetable juices and shred into salads.

Blackcurrants ~ Powerhouses of vitamin C and minerals. Tone and cleanse the blood. Make a syrup from the fresh berries and drink with pure spring water. Stew with other summer fruits.

Cinnamon ~ A delicious warming spice. Gently boosts blood circulation and tones the lungs. Sprinkle powdered cinnamon into breakfast cereals, and stew fruits like apple and pear with cinnamon sticks.

Ginger ~ Warms and stimulates blood flow to the extremities. Grate fresh root ginger into stir-fries and vegetable dishes. Use powdered ginger in baking and sweet puddings.

Ginkgo biloba (maidenhair) ~ Improves circulation all over the body. Contains flavonoids called ginkgolides that strengthen and protect the blood capillaries. May be helpful in shifting cellulite. Available in supplement form.

Ginseng ~ One of the so-called 'superior' Chinese medical herbs, ginseng is an adaptogen which ensures tissues receive enough oxygen in times of stress. Strengthens the heart and circulatory system, boosts energy and stamina. Sip three cups of Panax ginseng tea a day until your energy returns.

TOP TEN ENERGISING ESSENTIAL OILS

basil

ginger

grapefruit

lavender

lemon

nutmeg

orange

peppermint

rose

rosemary

Prunes and plums ~ Rich in iron and superb sources of lung-protecting antioxidants. Ideal for breakfasts, snacks and puddings.

Rosemary ~ An excellent tonic and all round stimulant. Warms and energises the body and strengthens the capillaries that feed the skin. Season dishes with fresh rosemary, sip infusions of the leaves and flowers.

Watercress ~ Rich in iron, vitamin C, folic acid, beta-carotene. Cleanses and fortifies the blood. Add small quantities to vegetable juice. Sprinkle in salads and add to soups.

Bath boost

Mix together 30g (1oz) each of lavender, thyme, marjoram, rosemary and peppermint, place in a muslin bag and hang from the bath taps to allow water to run over it. An ideal morning pick-me-up.

For face massage ~ 6 drops of essential oil in 30ml (2 tablespoons) of carrier oil.

For body massage ~ 12 drops of essential oil in 30ml (2 tablespoons) of carrier oil.

— *Recipes* —

INSTANT ENERGY BATH OIL

4 drops orange essential oil
4 drops basil essential oil
1 tablespoon organic milk

Dissolve the essential oils in a tablespoon of organic milk and add to a running bath.

WARM-UP BODY OIL

6 drops orange essential oil
4 drops nutmeg essential oil
2 drops ginger essential oil
30ml (2 tablespoons) sweet almond oil

Blend the essential oils with the almond oil. Ideal pre-exercise massage oil or for rubbing into the body after a warm bath or shower.

For an energising bath ~ Dissolve 10 drops of your chosen essential oil in a tablespoon of organic milk and add to the bath.

֍ Energise in the morning to wake your body up and whenever you are in the need of a vitality boost.

smooth

CHAPTER SIX

Refining

~

The Essence of Smoothness

Perfect skin is smooth and firm. These are youthful qualities which are an outer reflection of sleek muscles and a free flowing lymph system. Yet they are not ruled by the passage of time – even a young skin can appear puffy and ill-defined. When sleek contours give way to sagging and sponginess it's a sure sign of inner congestion and lack of muscle tone. Treatments aimed to free the flow of lymph, refine the muscles and tone-up the skin can roll back the years.

Be refined.

High Definition

While softness is superficial, skin's smoothness is defined
at a deeper level.

Lying beneath the epidermis is the dermal layer which gives skin its spring and suppleness. The dermis is intimately connected to the subcutaneous fatty cells and muscle fibres. These three structures together determine how firm and well-defined our skin looks and feels from the outside.

Good muscle tone gives skin definition. When the muscles grow flaccid from under use, the skin that lies over them begins to sag, irrespective of its age. The most effective way to give the face and body a natural lift is by toning up the muscles. Exercises which stretch and lengthen muscles as they work help to cultivate smooth, sleek contours.

The fatty layer provides a padding which makes skin feel soft and sensuous. While most women are preoccupied with whittling away excess fat cells, it is worth remembering that dieting is unselective. Cutting back on calories will not necessarily shift fat from where we would like – namely the hips, tummy, bottom and thighs. This is because fat metabolism is complex and various other factors come into play.

The female hormone, oestrogen, is primarily responsible for cultivating feminine curves. It appears to hold sway over the distribution of fatty tissue and needs to be taken into account when we set about remodelling our physique.

REFINING FORCE

The skin, fatty tissue and muscles are richly supplied with blood capillaries that feed them with oxygen and nutrients. They are also bathed in a clear fluid that leaches from the walls of these tiny vessels. This liquid is known as lymph and it is similar to blood in every way except it has no red cells. Most of us know little about the lymphatic system, but it holds the key to smoother, firmer skin and enhanced health.

Lymph's purpose is to pick up any cellular by-products that are too large to pass into the blood capillaries and whisk them away so the tissues don't become congested with their own wastes. When the lymph flows smoothly, the skin feels smooth and firm. But if the lymph laden with wastes lingers in the underlying tissues, the skin starts to look puffy and swollen.

INVISIBLE NETWORK

Although its primary role is deep-tissue cleansing, the lymphatic system is also part of the circulatory and immune system.

The lymph vessels form an intricate network of channels that spread throughout the body. Having cleared cells of debris (which may include old cells, bacteria and toxins), the lymph drains away from the tissues and flows along the thin-walled lymphatic canals towards the heart.

On its journey this opaque fluid passes through lymph nodes which feel like small nodules. Found under the chin, in the armpits, behind the knees and in the groin, the lymph nodes are like clearing stations. They contain large numbers of white blood cells or lymphocytes capable of engulfing noxious substances including bacteria and viral cells. Here lymph is cleaned and purified before being returned to the bloodstream at a junction in the upper thorax beneath the collar bone.

Every day 2 litres (3½ pints) of cleansed lymph is returned to the bloodstream.

SYSTEM OVERLOAD

The lymph system is most efficient when doing simple day-to-day cleansing duties. But any kind of infection, such as a cold or the flu, more than doubles its daily work-load. When the nodes feel tender or swollen it shows the lymph system is working overtime. As the lymph clears away all kinds of impurities, the more rubbish we take in the harder it must work.

Over-exposure to environmental pollutants such as air pollutants, impurities in water and pesticides sprayed on food crops, coupled with drinking too much alcohol and coffee, and eating lots of refined, starchy foods laden with additives can overload the lymphatic system. When the lymph is burdened with external toxins it cannot perform its normal cleansing activities so effectively. As impurities accumulate, the underlying tissues get congested and the skin becomes puffy and prone to painful spots. If nothing is done to cleanse the lymph and get it flowing freely, the conditions are perfect for the onset of cellulite in certain areas.

Signs of congestion include:

under-eye puffiness

pasty complexion

painful spots

frequent colds and infections

spongy-textured skin

persistent sinusitis

recurrent catarrh

cellulite

— Body brushing —

Brushing the skin with a natural-bristle brush is one of the most effective ways to get the lymph fluid moving. There are other benefits, too. Brushing removes dead cells and other impurities which increases the skin's capacity for elimination. It also stimulates the circulation to oxygenate the skin cells and improves muscle tone. Five minutes of energetic skin brushing is reputedly as effective at enhancing physical tone as 30 minutes of jogging.

- Invest in a natural-bristle brush (preferably one made with Mexican tampico fibres), with a long, detachable handle.
- Before showering or bathing, give your body a 5-minute, intense body brush.
- Always work towards the heart using long, smooth strokes.
- Start at the soles of the feet and brush up the legs and thighs towards the lymph nodes in the groin. Work in circular clockwise movements over the tummy (5–10 times).
- Brush over the hands and up the arms to the shoulders. Use the handle to brush upwards over the bottom, up the back and then across the top of the shoulders.
- Use downward strokes on the neck, throat and over the chest.

SPRING CLEANING

Blood circulation is powered by the heart, but the lymph has no such driving force. Its flow relies on the gentle squeezing brought about by deep rhythmic breathing and the contractions of major muscle groups. Moving, deep breathing and regular exercise are the best ways to keep lymph flowing freely.

However, there will be times when your lymph system needs a little extra help to clear away any congestion.

It is especially beneficial to do a lymph 'spring-clean' sometime during February or March to help it shake off the residues of winter coughs and colds. This will help to tone, firm and smooth skin in time for summer.

Manual Lymphatic Drainage

This is a powerful tissue-cleansing treatment given by a specially
trained therapist who has a sound knowledge of the lymphatic network.

Unlike traditional massage, this treatment uses the lightest finger pressure to stroke lymph in the right direction and so helps clear areas of congestion and stagnation. It works wonders for toning and refining skin all over the body, as well as for removing dark circles and puffiness under the eyes. Lymph drainage for the face is like having a mini facelift. This treatment is most effective in the hands of a professional, but there are a few helpful movements you can try. Always use a featherweight touch. Applying too much pressure may impede lymph flow.

- Using the fingertips, stroke down the cheeks close to the ears. You may even feel slight swelling or nodules under the skin close to the ear lobes. Gently coax the lymph down towards the nodes in the neck.
- From the shoulder blades stroke down and in towards the heart. Use the right hand to massage the left side and vice versa.
- Stimulate the lymph glands under the arms with a gentle squeezing action. With your right hand place the thumb under the left clavicle (collar) bone and clasp the pectoral muscle with your fingers. Squeeze and release about 10 times. Do the same on the other side.
- With light fingertip pressure gently massage the lymph nodes behind the knees. Always work in an upwards direction, from the calves to the thighs.
- Cold blast – Alternate warm and cold showers are not only great circulation boosters, they also get the lymph moving too. Take a warm shower for 2–3 minutes first, then switch to cold for about 20 seconds. A good time to do this is after body brushing.
- Feet treat – In reflexology the lymphatic system is mapped out on the surface of the foot and around the ankles. A good way to get at the lymph is to massage the feet. Add about 4 drops of a decongesting essential oil like lemon or peppermint to a tablespoon of carrier oil. Massage all over the feet, then start working on the lymph reflexes. Work your fingers from the tip of the toes up towards the ankle. Pay special attention to the webbing between the toes. Now work around the ankles themselves.

Refining and Firming Plants

Plants offer a two-pronged approach for smoothing the skin.

From the inside, certain plant foods help to cleanse the lymph and boost the body's natural immunity. When the infection-fighting force works well, the lymphatic system is free to go about its daily cleansing duties. From the outside, plant extracts help to tone the skin while antiseptic essential oils keep infections at bay.

FROM WITHIN

Garlic and onions ~ These pungent plants are both rich in sulphur compounds that are naturally antibiotic. As well as warding off bacteria, they boost the immune response to help shake off infections. Eaten on a regular basis they help to cleanse the lymph and blood.

Shiitake mushrooms ~ Highly regarded in Traditional Chinese Medicine for their immune-boosting properties. Add them to stews, stir-fries and soups to keep infections at bay. (Some people find mushrooms difficult to digest. If you suffer extreme bloating and wind after eating them, choose another option.) The recommended intake is one or two a day.

Wheatgrass juice ~ An excellent lymph cleanser. Whenever skin starts to look congested try to drink a 25ml (1fl oz) shot of pure wheatgrass juice each day or dilute with fresh carrot juice.

Echinacea ~ Otherwise known as purple cone flower, this herb gives the immune system extra impetus for fighting infections. Echinacea is a powerful lymph purifier and is very effective for refining the skin and clearing away blemishes.

Avoid taking echinacea continuously. It works best as a short sharp boost. Take 15–20 drops of tincture in water for up to ten days.

> **TOP TEN LYMPH-PURIFYING ESSENTIAL OILS**
>
> basil
> grapefruit
> juniper
> lemon
> orange
> peppermint
> pettigrain
> rosemary
> tea tree
> thyme

Horsetail ~ This weedy-looking herb is a rich source of silica and is the number one herb used in cosmetic preparations aimed at firming and toning the skin.

Make an infusion by simmering 30g (1oz) of herb in 570ml (1 pint) of water and sip from time to time if you can bear the taste. If not, wrap the herb in muslin (or use a horsetail tea bag) and leave to steep in the bath. Use body-toning preparations containing horsetail.

Other skin-refining herbs are **butcher's broom**, **meadowsweet**, **horse chestnut** and **ginseng**. Try adding a few drops of their tinctures to your favourite body lotion.

- Add a few drops of your favourite essential oil to a nighttime bath or add 4–6 drops to a tablespoon of carrier oil and smooth into the body, working in the direction of lymph flow, after showering or bathing.

- Use toning treatments every morning and every evening whenever your skin is in need of refining. Good for the summer months when skin is on display.

— *Recipe* —

LEMON REFINING LOTION
(for all-over toning and firming)

1 tablespoon aloe vera gel
2 tablespoons horsetail infusion
20 drops horse-chestnut tincture
4 drops lemon essential oil
4 drops peppermint essential oil

Spoon the aloe vera gel into a small bowl then stir in the horsetail infusion. When well blended add in the horse-chestnut tincture and essential oils.

Smooth this refreshing gel into the skin, working in the direction of lymph flow. For maximum benefits, first brush the skin and then shower before applying this gel all over.

Keeps up to a week when chilled.

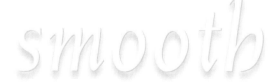

Body Specifics

Skin all over the body benefits from contouring treatments.
However, some areas need more attention than others to keep the skin
firm, smooth and well toned.

BEAUTIFUL BREASTS

Like any part of the body, our breasts respond to tender loving care. Treatments cannot perform miracles, but they can go a long way towards preserving skin's youthful definition.

Breast tissue is made up of two-thirds fatty tissue. While changes in weight do affect breast size, the female hormones – especially oestrogen – also influence how full they are. Breast size can increase a cup size or more during pregnancy.

Breasts have little natural support. With no muscles of their own they rely instead on the pectoral muscles attached to the chest and the weedier muscles of the neck which fan out across the cleavage. When these muscles are well toned the breasts are held firmly in place. When neglected they allow the bust to sag. No treatment cream or gel can compensate for poor muscle tone. And although wearing a bra makes the muscles redundant, the relentless pull of gravity is far more damaging.

Natural uplift

Spray the breasts with cold water at the end of a bath or shower. With the shower attachment work in small circular movements giving each breast a short 30- to 60-second cold blast. Alternatively try crushing up ice and wrapping it in a flannel or some muslin to form a compress. Cover each breast with this ice mask for a few minutes.

Certain plants and foods contain chemicals which are structurally very similar to oestrogen, the hormone that enhances the shape and firmness of breasts. These phyto-oestrogens are weaker than those the body makes but eating foods such as soya and flax seeds which are rich in these substance, and using preparations rich in phyto-oestrogenic plants like hops, sage and fennel, may help to keep your breasts well toned.

— Recipes —

UPLIFTING GEL
(for the bust)

1 tablespoon aloe vera gel

1 tablespoon horsetail infusion

10 drops hops tincture

4 drops lemon essential oil

4 drops geranium essential oil

Spoon the aloe vera gel into a small glass dish. Stir in the horsetail infusion, then add in the drops of hops and the essential oils. Blend together. Decant into a small glass jar and smooth on first thing every morning and evening. Keeps up to a week when chilled.

CONTOUR SMOOTHING MASSAGE OIL

30ml (2 tablespoons) soya oil

4 drops rosemary essential oil

4 drops lavender essential oil

2 drops lemon essential oil

2 drops juniper essential oil

Pour the soya oil into a small dish and add the essential oils. Decant into a small, tinted glass bottle. Massage into cellulite-prone areas, ideally after body brushing and a warm bath. You can also add these essences to your bath to enhance the effects. Keeps fresh for up to 6 months.

— To keep the breasts pert, you should work these muscles every day —

1. Press your hands together in front of your chest, as if praying, and push as hard as possible for 10 seconds.

2. Hold your arms out to the sides, with fists clenched, at shoulder height and circle forwards 10 times, then backwards 10 times.

3. Adopt the press-up position. Bend your arms slightly to lower the body (not all the way to the ground) and straighten them again. Do this 10 times.

4. Do the breaststroke (as in swimming), preferably in water as it offers more resistance than air. Cold water also tightens the tissues.

5. Grimace, to work the neck muscles.

BEAUTIFUL BEHIND

Most women are unhappy with their bottom and upper thighs. This is because the skin here is particularly prone to sponginess. We call this orange-peel effect 'cellulite' but its existence is cloaked in controversy. From the medical viewpoint the skin's bumpy texture is blamed on the underlying fat cells. But if this is so, why aren't other padded areas such as the tummy and upper arms bumpy too.

The feminine hormone oestrogen seems partly to blame. As well as favouring the accumulation of fat in these areas, this hormone encourages fluid retention so the tissues are easily water-logged. This makes skin feel spongy.

Stress and inactivity make matters worse. Muscles that are tense or under-worked impede the smooth flow of blood and lymph. When this happens the fat cells become starved of oxygen and blood while wastes accumulate in the underlying tissues. These toxins irritate collagen fibrils and in time they wrap themselves around fat cells. These fatty nodules can be felt as tiny lumps beneath the skin in the most advanced stages of cellulite.

Many factors contribute to creating cellulite. The best way to keep skin in this area smooth and sleek is to eliminate as many of them as possible.

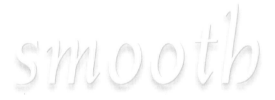

– Beat cellulite –

❧ Work the muscles. Sitting for long periods at a time means the muscles in this area don't do much work. If you work behind a desk, get up every half an hour and walk around. Walking up stairs is good exercise for the bottom and leg muscles. When muscles are active they burn up excess fat stores around them.

❧ Brush the body. Stimulating these areas helps to boost both blood flow and lymph drainage.

❧ Squeeze it. A stimulating massage involving movements like squeezing and pummelling release tension from muscles, boost blood circulation and move fluids from the tissues to prevent cellulite from settling in.

❧ Spray it away. Spraying the hips, bottom and thighs with jets of warm and cold water works wonders for revving up the circulation. Drink plenty of pure spring water – it helps flush fluids out of the tissues.

❧ Boost metabolism. Many plants contain mild stimulants that give metabolism a boost and so help to prevent fat from accumulating in the tissues. Recent research suggests Japanese green tea helps to burn off excess fat. Try drinking green tea each day.

❧ Strengthen the capillaries. Keeping the tiny blood capillaries in good shape helps blood to flow freely to the fat cells and prevents cellulite from forming. Seek out foods rich in capillary protecting antioxidants such as the plant-derived anthocyanidins present in blue-purple berry fruits like bilberries, blueberries, cherries and black grapes. The odd glass of antioxidant-rich red wine is fine, but avoid caffeine which tends to restrict blood flow.

❧ Use plant refiners. Massaging cellulite-prone areas with an oil containing stimulating, cleansing, diuretic and refining essential oils on a regular basis will keep the contours sleek and smooth.

serenity

CHAPTER SEVEN

De-stressing

~

The Essence of Serenity

Stress is skin's arch enemy. Yet, for many of us, anxiety and worry are an everyday part of life. Feeling frazzled can bring on skin problems from an oil crisis to over-sensitivity. Stress and strain become etched on the skin as wrinkles. Relaxation and soothing massage strokes work together with calming herbs and essential oils to melt away the angst. De-stressing will rebalance and rejuvenate your skin, so let go.

Be at peace.

The Nature of Stress

Stress comes in different guises and what is stressful to you will not necessarily bother someone else. However, we all experience stress in the same way.

When something makes us feel anxious, nervous, frightened or even excited our adrenal glands start to pump out adrenaline. This is the number one stress hormone. Adrenaline speeds up our heart beat, breathing and metabolic rate to give us a rush of extra energy.

The stress reaction is designed for survival. In earlier times, when stress came in the form of man-eating tigers or hostile tribes, the energy surge was essential for fighting or fleeing. We tend to see stress as being negative, but it can still be beneficial. Adrenaline provides an exhilarating buzz that motivates and energises. Stress enhances our capacity to cope so we are better prepared to deal with the next crisis that comes along. But for stress to be healthy we must be free to relax and regain our sense of balance before the next challenge arises.

Nowadays our stresses are different from those experienced by our ancestors and, while rarely life-threatening, are almost ever-present. Modern sources of stress include being late for work, failing an exam, getting an unexpected bill or losing our job. When stuck in traffic, fighting or running away is useless so the energy surge has no outlet. Instead it gets bottled up and we end up feeling frustrated, angry and irritable. As stress is often experienced day after day there is never time to unwind and re-centre ourselves.

Continuous surges of adrenaline and over-stimulation of the nervous system bombard the body with stress chemicals. When constantly anxious and on edge, our muscles tense and we end up feeling fatigued. Relentless and ongoing stress eventually brings burn-out.

STRESSING THE SKIN

Stress affects our skin in a variety of different ways. Here's how:

- Adrenaline redirects blood away from the skin and sends it to the muscles instead. This is the reason skin becomes pale and washed out after a sudden shock, or during times of relentless stress and strain.

- Anger, irritability, excitement and frustration

unleash chemicals which goad the sebaceous glands into pouring out more oil. The excess sebum can block the pores and encourage pimples to form. This is why we tend to break out in spots on the eve of an important occasion.

- Chronic stress makes muscles tense up and become stiff. This prevents the free flow of blood bearing oxygen and vital nutrients to the skin. Tension also hinders the swift removal of wastes from the underlying tissue. This explains why stressed skin lacks vitality and looks congested. Over the years tension becomes etched on our faces, hence the term 'worry lines'.

- Strain slows down the rate of cell turnover so the fresh epidermal cells take longer to reach the surface. By the time they get there, much of their moisture has disappeared. As a result skin looks dull and sallow when we are under constant pressure.

- Persistent stress results in the secretion of cortisol which suppresses the body's natural immunity. When skin is stressed from within its resilience crumbles and it is more likely to react to potential irritants such as perfume. The best way to prevent over-sensitivity is to de-stress your skin.

– Mini meditation –

Allowing yourself to withdraw from the outside world for 10–15 minutes a day will help you find inner stillness. Meditation is a way of focusing the mind to clear away the clutter. You can silently recite a one word 'mantra' or do this simple exercise.

- Dim the lights or draw the curtains, then light a candle. With legs crossed, sit on the floor with the candle in front of you. Watch the flame dance before your eyes. Hold your gaze until the image appears hazy then slowly close your eyes. Try to keep the flame in your mind's eye. If your thoughts start to wander, open your eyes slightly to recapture the image and begin again.

- True beauty is an outer reflection of inner peace and self-confidence. On a psychological level stress shatters serenity and fuels self-doubt. You can lavish care and attention on your skin but unless you feel composed and enjoy a sense of self-worth, the beauty you desire will always lie just out of reach.

Pathways to Peace

Is life so full of stress you've forgotten what it feels like to be truly
relaxed and at peace with the world?

It's easy to become addicted to being stressed. Rushing around makes us feel busy and industrious. To take things at a more relaxed pace can seem lazy and irresponsible. But this is a myth. In reality, relaxation lifts tiredness and sets our energy free. When our mind is still and clear of internal chatter, it is easier to think clearly and make decisions. Being at peace sharpens our intuition so we instinctively know what is best for us. Life flows better when we let go a little.

Being relaxed reverses the damage stress does to our skin, too. When our body settles into a state of balance, skin starts to behave normally. Problems we assume are part of our make-up often disappear.

As tension melts from the muscles, deep lines and wrinkles are soothed away. This explains why we often look and feel ten years younger after a relaxing holiday. Serenity shines through our skin.

Cast your mind back to a time – a special holiday for example – when you managed to break free from the endless cycle of stress. Remember how it felt to be released from the tug

of time. Now try to imagine how different life would be if you could always feel this way.

Such inner tranquillity lies within everyone's grasp. The path to peace lies in taking every opportunity to nip stress in the bud before it has a chance to become ingrained in your life.

Techniques for relaxation

Discovering the art of relaxation brings balance back into your life. There are a number of tried and tested ways for letting go of tension. You may have already tried the Mini meditation on page 99. Here are some other techniques. The best are the simplest and are easy to squeeze into a hectic schedule.

Visualisation ~ Letting your imagination run free is a good way to unwind. Visualisation techniques are essentially day-dreaming with one restriction – don't allow anyone else into your dream world as it will break the spell.

 ♦ Find a place where you are not going to be distracted – take the phone off the hook, turn off the fax and switch on the answering machine. Settle into a comfortable chair and close your eyes. Mentally transport yourself to a place (either real or imaginary) that makes you feel happy and relaxed. It may be a sandy white beach lapped by azure waves or a field of vibrant sunflowers. Make your paradise come alive. Imagine the sun's warmth or a balmy breeze brushing against your skin. Sink deeper and deeper into the stillness. Stay there for between 15–20 minutes, then slowly open your eyes and return to the real world.

Soothing strokes ~ Massage is one of the most effective anti-stress treatments. Its smooth, sweeping strokes and gentle finger pressure work wonders for soothing the psyche and promoting deep relaxation. On a psychological level massage provides the comfort we crave in troubled times. The lightest touch provides reassurance and raises self-esteem. On a physical level it coaxes tension from muscles and revitalises the circulation.

While a one-hour face and body massage relieves anxiety as effectively as any 30-minute exercise regime, to nip stress in the bud it is a good idea to have treatments on a regular basis – ideally once a week or fortnight. Giving a massage to a friend or partner is also a very good way of dispelling stress and will leave you feeling relaxed as well.

Certain massage movements work wonders for bringing almost instant calm.

- Stroking, slowly and rhythmically down the back over and over again is wonderfully soporific.

- Pressuring, using the balls of the thumbs and fingerpads to needle away at knotty areas, is the basis of a shiatsu-style massage renowned for its stress-busting powers. Work over the shoulders and upper back.

- Using the fingertips to work over the scalp and neck area can bring deep relaxation in a matter of minutes.

Supreme stress buster ~ Stress turns sour when there is no vent for our adrenaline-fuelled energy rush. Exercise is the ideal substitute for fighting or fleeing. As stress chemicals accumulate in the body, skin often breaks out in spots or looks pale and washed out.

- If feeling frustrated and angry, the more vigorous kinds of activity such as aerobic work-outs, kick-boxing or tae bo and ashtanga yoga will discharge your pent-up energy.

- If feeling worn out by strain, the gentler forms of exercise like walking, swimming, sivananda yoga, tai chi and pilates will restore your natural vitality.

Anti-stress Diet

The sort of food you eat can either help to instil a sense of calmness
and balance, or make you feel even more anxious and at sea.

FOODS THAT SOOTHE

Almonds ~ These nuts contain magnesium, a mineral sometimes known as nature's tranquil-liser. It helps to keep the nerves on an even keel. Nibbling these nuts between meals instead of sweet snacks stabilises blood sugars and helps to keep energy levels steady.

Bananas ~ A rich source of tryptophan, an amino acid that we convert into serotonin. Serotonin is a brain chemical associated with feeling calm and content. Anxiety, depression and stress-induced insomnia are linked to low levels of this chemical. Other foods containing pre-formed serotonin are dates, red and blue plums, aubergines, papaya, passion fruit, pineapple and tomatoes.

Figs ~ One of the best plant sources of calcium, a mineral which helps to relax the muscles. Low levels of calcium are linked to anxiety and nervousness. Other good sources are chickpeas, natural yoghurt, green leafy vegetables and shellfish.

Flax oil ~ The richest natural source of omega 3 fatty acids which are needed to make healthy brain and nervous tissue. They also keep the skin soft and smooth. These fatty acids are also present in soya beans, walnuts and pumpkin seeds, as well as oily fish such as salmon and mackerel.

Wholegrains ~ These provide plenty of B vitamins which are needed to soothe and strengthen the nerves. B vitamins are rapidly depleted by stress. As they cannot be stored in the body we need a good supply every day. They help to keep blood sugar levels stable and provide a steady source of energy. Good sources are brown rice, wheat, rye and oats.

FOODS THAT FRAZZLE

Biscuits, cakes and pastries ~ These are made from refined (white) sugar and flour which are depleted of B vitamins. Like adrenaline they give a sudden rush of energy which quickly wears off. What the body needs in times of stress is a slow and steady supply of energy.

Red meat ~ This is rich in tyrosine, an amino acid which the body converts to adrenaline. On the plus side it can make you feel more alert and energised, but if you are already on edge it will exacerbate feelings of agitation. Tyrosine is also present in eggs and cheese.

Chocolate ~ Rich in sugar and a mild stimulant known as theobromine, this number one comfort food can actually enhance feelings of anxiety and irritability. If you can't resist, opt instead for dark chocolate (90 per cent cocoa butter) which is rich in soothing magnesium.

Coffee ~ Three cups of coffee can raise adrenaline levels by 200 per cent. This is because coffee goads the adrenal glands into producing adrenaline when it isn't genuinely needed.

NATURE'S TRANQUILLISERS

Certain plants and herbs help to boost your natural resistance to life's ups and downs.

Avena Sativa ~ A tincture made from oats which helps to calm and strengthen the nervous system. Ideal for nervous exhaustion.

Camomile ~ This soothes the nervous system and is especially helpful for stomach upsets and cramps caused by stress. Make an infusion or take as a tincture.

Daminara ~ A Native American aphrodisiac excellent for relieving stress-induced anxiety, depression and loss of libido. Works by strengthening the nervous system to increase resilience to stress. Make an infusion or take as a tincture.

Kava kava ~ Acclaimed as nature's answer to Librium, kava has been used for centuries by native South Sea islanders who have been called the happiest people on earth. Kava induces relaxation and relieves feelings of anxiety without causing drowsiness. Available as a tincture or in tablet form.

Orange blossom ~ The heady scented blossom from the orange tree helps to ease anxiety and nervous depression. Dilute a little orange flower water with hot water to make a soothing drink. From these flowers comes the essential oil neroli with its tranquillising and slightly hypnotic perfume.

Passionflower (passiflora) ~ A sedative which brings deep relaxation. Good for nervous tension and when you feel on edge. Make an infusion or take as a tincture.

ESSENTIAL OILS

For face massage ~ Add 6 drops of essential oil to 30ml (2 tablespoons) of carrier oil.

For body massage ~ Add 12 drops of essential oil to 30ml (2 tablespoons) of carrier oil.

For a soothing bath ~ Add 10 drops of essential oil to a tablespoon of organic milk and add to the bath.

To create a peaceful atmosphere ~ Place a few drops of your favourite essential oil on to an aroma burner or drop into a bowl of just-boiled water. Frankincense and sandalwood are a wonderful aid to meditation.

FLORAL STRESS RELIEF

Flower remedies (also known as flower essences) are subtle elixirs that help to relieve the symptoms of stress. Different flowers, it seems, encapsulate the various emotions and feelings we experience. Remedies made from these flowers work by dissolving away the negative mind states which restores our sense of inner peace and emotional equilibrium. This floral therapy dates back to antiquity. Thousands of years ago Australian Aborigines and Native Americans used flowers to soothe turbulent emotions and achieve peace of mind.

The art of healing with flowers was rediscovered in the 1930s by Dr Edward Bach, a respected Harley Street physician who became increasingly dissatisfied with the orthodox approach to treating illness.

Bach became convinced that stress is a root cause of much ill health and that your personality influences your stress response and how you deal with life's dilemmas. In difficult times some people become irritable and angry, while others are more likely to become withdrawn or gloomy. He began to search for a new healing system that could help people to cope with stress in its many different guises, and he found it in flowers.

There are 12 Bach flower remedies that relate to 12 key personality types and a further 26

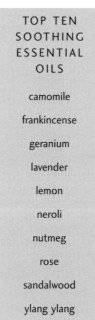

TOP TEN
SOOTHING
ESSENTIAL
OILS

camomile

frankincense

geranium

lavender

lemon

neroli

nutmeg

rose

sandalwood

ylang ylang

remedies for dealing with specific states of mind. Since Bach created his remedies, other flowers from across the world have been investigated and there are now hundreds of different remedies or essences to suit every conceivable state of being.

Flower remedies are the perfect complement to essential oils especially if they both come from the same source. For example, camomile flower remedy will add another dimension to the calming benefits of camomile essential oil.

FLORAL SKINCARE

Flower remedies can help to nip stress in the bud before it has a chance to play havoc with your skin. If you are already feeling frazzled, they will help to restore a sense of calm and equilibrium.

§ Choose one or two remedies that describe how you are feeling at this moment (see chart on page 106). Add 2 drops to a glass of pure spring water, juice or tisane, or drop directly under the tongue three times a day or, if in a state of shock, every hour until your composure returns.

– Recipe –
SOOTHING MASSAGE OIL
(for the face)

4 drops neroli essential oil

1 drop camomile essential oil

1 drop ylang ylang essential oil

10 drops of your chosen flower remedy

30ml (2 tablespoons) sweet almond oil

Blend the essential oils with the almond oil. Decant into a dark glass bottle. Use about a teaspoonful at a time. Massage for 5 minutes, tissue off and spray with floral water. For the body, add double the quantity of essential oils in the same amount of carrier oil. Keeps fresh for up to 6 months.

§ Another way to enjoy the benefits of flower remedies is to add them to the skin cream or lotion you use each day. There are several flower essence creams available to buy, but why not personalise your own moisturiser by stirring in a few drops of an appropriate flower remedy. Add approximately 10 drops to 15ml (1 tablespoon) of cream or lotion.

REMEDIES TO RESTORE INNER PEACE

How you feel	Helpful Flower Remedies
Angry	Holly (Bach Flower), Mountain Devil (Australian Bush), Orange-spiked Pea Flower (Australian Living)
Anxious	Filaree (Flower Essence Society), Purple Flag Flower (Australian Living), Red Chestnut (Bach Flower)
Exhausted	Banksia Robur (Australian Bush), Gorse (Findhorn), Indian Paintbrush (Flower Essence Society), Olive (Bach Flower)
Frustrated	Silver Princess Gum (Australian Living), Wild Oat (Bach Flower)
In shock	Arnica (Flower Essence Society), Fringed Violet (Australian Bush), Pear (Master's Flower Essences), Rescue Remedy (Bach Flower), Scottish Primrose (Findhorn), Star of Bethlehem (Bach Flower)
Irritable	Black-eyed Susan (Australian Bush), Impatiens (Bach Flower), Lettuce (Master's Flower Essences)
Lacking confidence	Kerato (Bach Flower), Five Corners (Australian Bush), Larch (Bach Flower), Pretty Face (Flower Essence Society)
Moody	Chamomile (Flower Essence Society), Peach-flowered Tea Tree (Australian Bush), Scleranthus (Bach Flower),
Unhappy	Cherry (Master's Flower Essences), Gorse (Bach Flower), Rhododendron (Deva Flower Elixirs), Sturt Desert Pea (Australian Bush), Valerian (Findhorn)
Worried	Brown Boronia (Australian Living), Crowea (Australian Bush), White Chestnut (Bach Flower)

Beauty Sleep
— The Ultimate Relaxation

Sleep is a time for deep relaxation and renewal.

While we slumber our skin is being repaired and regenerated. Nothing refreshes both mind and body quite like a good night's sleep. Every night we go through, four to six cycles of sleep, each lasting between 90 and 100 minutes.

As we drift into sleep our brainwaves slow right down and we enter the first phase known as non-rapid eye movement sleep. This is a quiet phase when the heart beat and breathing slow down. During this time the body's restorative processes kick in and go about repairing damaged tissues. There is a surge of growth hormone which stimulates cell renewal.

At the end of this deep sleep phase comes a period of rapid eye movement (REM) sleep during which we dream. The eyes flicker back and forth, blood supply to the brain increases, breathing speeds up and our temperature rises a little. This kind of sleep seems to be essential for discharging stress and lack of REM sleep may leave you feeling restless, anxious and over-excitable. During this time, memory retention and information organisation is taking place in the brain's higher centres. Periods of REM sleep seem to get longer when life is particularly demanding or stressful. Then the cycle starts over again. In total, sleep comprises 80 per cent deep and 20 per cent REM sleep.

HOW MANY WINKS?

Our sleep needs are highly individual and vary from day to day. After a particularly stressful or action-packed day you may need more sleep to recover. Most people feel refreshed and restored by seven to eight hours of sleep. Ironically the more stressed you are, the more elusive sleep can be.

If you find it difficult to drift off or wake up in the middle of the night, you may begin to feel tired, irritable, anxious and lack concentration the next day. The effects of sleep deprivation seem to be cumulative. The longer you suffer from sleeplessness, the more exhausted you feel.

There is some evidence to suggest lack of sleep also accelerates ageing which is bad news for our skin. The good news is we can catch up on sleep, so take every opportunity to steal 40 winks.

— *Slip into slumber* —

Dos

- Get more exercise during the day. It discharges the adrenaline which keeps you alert and wakeful.

- Take a warm bath before bedtime with soothing essential oils.

- Massage a little diluted neroli or sandalwood essential oil into your chest or sprinkle a few drops of pure essential oil on your pillow case.

- Sip a cup of soothing herbal tea made from tranquillising herbs like lime flowers, vervain, scullcap, camomile and passionflower.

- Place a few drops of mind-calming flower essences under your tongue an hour before bedtime – try white chestnut (Bach Flower), cHamomile (Flower Essence Society), lettuce (Master's Flower Essences), brown boronia (Australian Living).

- Eat plenty of bananas and other foods that help the body to make serotonin (see page 102).

Don'ts

- Try to sleep when you are not tired. Potter around doing some sort of relaxing activity or read instead.

- Eat a heavy meal in the evening.

- Drink stimulants such as coffee and cola drinks in the evening. While alcohol initially relaxes the body, it has a rebound effect and tends to wake you up in the middle of the night.

- Let night wakefulness become a habit as it will be much harder to break. Resist getting up and pacing around. It's better to shut your eyes and do a mini meditation (see page 99).

serenity

harmony

CHAPTER EIGHT

Hormones in Harmony

~

The Essence of Eternal Beauty

Hormones are the body's movers and shakers. When working in harmony they have a positive influence on our skin. If thrown off balance they can alter its behaviour. For women, hormonal upheavals are part and parcel of life. Understanding how hormones influence our skin helps us understand why it sometimes acts out of character. Certain plants and nutrients help to smooth the transitions and restore a sense of balance. When your hormones are in harmony, skin looks its best at every stage in life.

Be balanced.

The Nature of Hormones

Hormones are the body's chemical messengers and every moment of
our lives various different ones are circulating in our bloodstream.

They convey the sort of information that enables tissues to communicate with one another. This ensures everything runs smoothly and harmoniously.

On a daily basis, hormones influence various cycles and bodily rhythms such as sleeping and waking. A surge of cortisol hormones wakes us up in the morning while melantonin, a hormone secreted when darkness falls, brings on feelings of sleepiness. Hormones like adrenaline are only secreted in times of stress. Hormones concerned with growth and development come into play during certain phases in our lives. For women, the menstrual cycle is governed by a particular set of hormones which fluctuate on a regular and predictable basis. These hormones influence the behaviour and appearance of our skin.

BALANCING ACT

Hormones are made by endocrine glands and their secretions are in turn synchronised by a small gland called the pituitary, found at the base of the brain. The pituitary is often referred to as the master gland because it ensures the

hormones work in harmony. The pituitary relays messages to the other endocrine glands through its own set of hormones. It in turn takes orders from a higher region of the brain known as the hypothalamus. Like a control centre, the hypothalamus processes information coming in via the senses and from inside the body, then determines the best course of action. In this way sensations such as pleasure and pain can bring about subtle hormonal changes in the body. Soothing massage strokes have, for example, been found to boost levels of the female hormones oestrogen and progesterone.

The hypothalamus is highly sensitive to stress which explains how our hormones can go haywire when we are emotionally frazzled.

NATURAL RHYTHM

For women the rhythmic rise and fall of hormones involved in the menstrual cycle accompanies most of adult life. As these hormones have the power to influence moods, emotions and various bodily processes, including the behaviour of skin, it is helpful to know a little about them. The term 'menstrual' comes from the Latin word *mensis* meaning month and its earlier derivation, 'the moon'. As the female cycle spans roughly the same length of time as the moon's 28-day period of waxing and waning, there seems to be a sort of synchronicity between the two.

The female cycle

The pituitary glands set the menstrual cycle in motion by secreting follicle stimulating hormone (FSH). This hormone travels to the ovaries where it stimulates the development of an immature ovum or egg within a follicle. As the ovum matures its follicle secretes a hormone known as oestrogen which causes the lining of the womb (uterus) to thicken.

At mid-cycle (around day 14) the oestrogen level peaks and the pituitary gland responds by sending out another hormone called luteinizing hormone (LH).

On reaching the ovaries, LH triggers the ovum to be released from its follicle. This is known as ovulation. As the mature ovum begins its journey down the fallopian tubes towards the womb the empty follicle, now called the corpus luteum, produces another hormone called progesterone as well as oestrogen. Under progesterone's influence, the uterus lining

becomes enriched with tiny blood vessels in preparation to receive the egg should it become fertilised. If the egg remains unfertilised, the corpus luteum shrivels up and stops producing progesterone. Levels of progesterone and oestrogen now plummet and cause the lining of the uterus to be shed. This marks the beginning of a period. About two days later the pituitary produces another surge of FSH and the cycle begins again.

Go with the flow

You will notice that your skin's behaviour changes subtly throughout the cycle. It tends to be more receptive at around mid-cycle, making this a good time for nourishing and replenishing treatments. In the days before your period is due your skin may be slightly oilier than usual. Now is the time to step up gentle exfoliation so as to prevent clogged pores and spots.

Digestion is often less efficient at this time so it is a good idea to eat simple meals prepared with lots of digestion-enhancing herbs such as sage, basil, rosemary, thyme and parsley. This will ensure your skin receives a good supply of essential nutrients. If your skin starts looking puffy prior to menstruation be sure to eat plenty of fluid-flushing foods such as celery, fennel and dandelion leaves.

Menstruation or bleeding is a time of elimination so this is a good time to cleanse the skin from within. Eat lightly and drink plenty of fresh fruit and vegetable juices during the first few days of a period.

HORMONAL UPHEAVAL

There are certain times in life when hormonal disturbances are predictable – at puberty, during pregnancy and at the menopause. However, various other factors can disrupt the cyclic flow of the female hormones and lead to imbalances in oestrogen and progesterone. These hormonal disruptions may cause our skin to act out of character and can be an underlying cause of problems such as sudden outbreaks of spots, excess oiliness or dryness, and the appearance of cellulite.

Luckily there are ways to restore hormonal harmony and bring the skin back into balance, as you'll see later in this chapter.

FERTILITY RITES

Most children are blessed with soft, flawless skin but this often changes with the onset of puberty. For both sexes this passage into adulthood is a time of hormonal flux which alters skin's nature and behaviour. At around the age of 12–13 (or 15 in boys) the hypothalamus releases a growth hormone which tells the pituitary to activate the reproductive organs.

In girls, the pituitary starts to secrete follicle stimulating hormone (FSH) which activates the ovaries. In boys, the very same hormone is known as interstitial cell stimulating hormone (ICSH) and it acts on the testes.

In the early days, menstrual cycles tend to be irregular and unpredictable, often occurring without ovulation. It may take a year for hormones to reach levels high enough to stimulate the monthly development of follicles and establish regular menstrual cycles.

TIME OF CHANGE

Oestrogen produced by the ovaries is responsible for cultivating curves. It stimulates breast tissue development and encourages the laying down of fat on hips, bottom and thighs. In an attempt to curb these physical changes, girls often resort to dieting. But cutting calories may also deprive skin of the nutrients it needs to look its best. A lack of vitamin A (or beta-carotene) may lead to blocked pores and pimples, while insufficient B vitamins encourage greasiness. Although testosterone is a predominantly male hormone, during adolescence levels rise in both boys and girls (to a lesser degree). This dynamising androgenic hormone fuels sex drive and may

– Ride the storm –

❧ Develop a good cleansing routine. It's essential to clear away excess oil. Don't resort to oil-stripping cleansers and toners as they may actually aggravate the sebaceous glands even more. Choose a gentle cleanser designed for oily skins such as a foaming wash or milk and use it as often as required. If your skin is spotty, choose one with tea tree essential oil, a mild anti-bacterial and healing agent. (See page 115 for more information on dealing with blackheads and spots.)

❧ Keep it simple. If your skin is oily it may not need a creamy moisturiser. For a refreshing moisture surge apply pure aloe vera gel. To help purify the pores add a few drops of lemon or lavender essential oil to a teaspoon of gel.

❧ Nourish yourself. If you want to stay slim and be kind to your skin eat masses of fresh fruits and vegetables. They are low in calories but packed with essential skin nutrients. If anything, ditch the junk food, biscuits and chocolate.

❧ Shed the stress. Find a way to discharge excess adrenaline so channelling aggression and rebalancing your emotions. Vigorous activities such as sport, aerobics, rowing and cycling are good. If you feel insecure and vulnerable, a good chat with a close friend is more helpful. The Bach flower remedy crab apple is helpful when you are feeling ugly and unhappy with who you are.

❧ At the end of a stressful day treat yourself to a long, languid bath with soothing essences such as neroli and camomile.

trigger feelings of anger and aggression. It also stimulates the sebaceous glands to produce sebum. When oily secretions increase, the scene is set for blocked pores and pimples. No wonder puberty is such a turbulent time.

These changes are a source of stress. Exam pressures and shifting social dynamics both at home and in school or college add to the load, making the teenage years a particularly stressful time of life.

Anxiety about skin problems also helps to set up a vicious circle. The more you worry about your skin, the worse it becomes. Take heart. The hormonal hell won't last forever and there are ways to smooth its passage.

Cycle of Life

Throughout our twenties, thirties and forties we expect our menstrual cycles
to run smoothly and regularly, but, in reality, hiccups frequently occur.

Hormone balance is a fragile affair and anything that upsets or confuses the hypothalamus has a knock-on effect. Like throwing a pebble into a still pond, it sends ripples through the body.

DISRUPTIVE INFLUENCES

Stress ~ This can overwhelm the hypothalamus which in turn sends mixed messages to the pituitary. A sudden shock can be responsible for a missed period. Similarly long-term pressure can disrupt the cycle and make periods unpredictable.

Dieting ~ The body interprets severe calorie restriction as starvation and rapid weight loss may result in a temporary shut-down of ovulation and menstruation which means hormone levels will plummet.

Lack of nutrients ~ A number of vitamins and minerals are involved in making hormones. The adrenal glands, for example, require vitamin C and pantothenic acid (vitamin B5) to produce adrenaline. Both oestrogen and progesterone are made from cholesterol in steps involving enzymes dependent on certain vitamins and minerals, especially vitamin B6 and magnesium.

Over-exercising ~ Female athletes undergoing intensive training often have irregular periods. Building up muscle and reducing fatty tissue to a minimum may be perceived by the body in the same way as dieting. Even if cycles are regular, ovulation may be skipped and progesterone levels will fall.

Illness ~ Hormone balance is often disrupted when the immune system is fighting off a viral or bacterial infection. A traumatic injury may also throw the cycles out of sync.

Pollutants ~ A number of man-made chemicals, known as xeno-oestrogens, have oestrogenic properties and seem capable of disrupting hormone balance. They appear to interfere with systems that regulate production of hormones, including oestrogen. Sources include organochlorine pesticides, fungicides, plastics, household cleaners and petrochemical derivatives such as mineral oil (present in many moisturisers and cosmetic preparations).

Circadian chaos ~ Anything that upsets the internal body clock, such as jet-lag and working night-shifts, tends to disrupt menstrual cycles. Air hostesses frequently skip periods as a result of crossing several time zones on long-haul flights. It can take two weeks for the body to re-establish normal rhythms after a single trans-Atlantic journey.

OUT OF BALANCE

Period problems are a tell-tale sign of hormone imbalance. If your periods are irregular, heavy and painful, or if you usually feel anxious and uncomfortable during the days leading up to a period, your hormones may well be out of kilter. This sets the scene for skin problems.

Pre-menstrual crisis ~ Many women (around 70 per cent) experience a range of uncomfortable symptoms prior to a period. Typical pre-menstrual symptoms include feeling irritable, depressed and insecure as well as cravings for sweets, tender breasts and headaches. At the same time skin acts out of character. The sebaceous glands can go into overdrive, making

pores appear larger and making conditions perfect for spots to form. Skin is inclined to be more sensitive and reactive at this time. Fluid retention makes the skin on hips and thighs spongy, and cellulite more obvious. The problems seem to be due to oestrogen levels remaining unusually high while progesterone falls.

Heavy and painful periods ~ These seem to be rooted in hormonal upsets and may indicate a problem with the thyroid gland. Excessive loss of blood can drain colour from the skin and leave it looking pale and lifeless. It is important to eat plenty of blood-building foods rich in iron, folic acid and vitamin B12 to ensure the skin receives enough oxygen and nutrients.

Irregular or skipped periods ~ These are usually caused by sudden shock or excessive long-term stress, rapid weight loss or over-exercising (unless pregnancy is a possibility). When periods are erratic the hormones are invariably out of sync. Skin behaves unpredictably at these times making it difficult to know whether to classify it as oily, combination or even dry as it may fluctuate. While restoring a sense of balance, it is important to be flexible and go with your skin's needs.

Re-synchronise

When steps are taken to soothe the hypothalamus and restore hormonal balance, period problems and their accompanying skin troubles invariably improve and in time may disappear.

Deal with the stress. Emotional upheavals and stress often lie at the root of hormonal problems. Flower remedies may be helpful here. Pomegranate (Flower Essence Society, Deva Flower Elixirs) and Quince (Deva) can help with the conflicts of juggling a family and career; She Oak (Australian Bush) can help with hormonal imbalances related to pre-menstrual tension.

Nourish yourself. Certain nutrients are involved in the pathways of hormone production. Vitamin B6 and magnesium are essential for making progesterone. Other key nutrients involved in hormone balance are zinc and the essential fatty acids.

Be predictable. Regular eating, sleeping and exercise patterns seem to encourage hormone

– Cut out chemicals –

If your hormones are out of balance, the last thing your body needs are chemicals that aggravate the oestrogenic effect. Although xeno-oestrogens crop up everywhere, it is possible to minimise your exposure to them. Here's how:

1. Use skincare preparations made from natural plant ingredients (preferably home-made), choose your make-up with care.

2. Avoid ready prepared microwave dishes (xeno-oestrogens leach from plastic when heated).

3. Don't wrap left-over food in clingfilm.

4. Never leave mineral water in plastic bottles in the sun.

5. Avoid spraying weed-killers and pesticides in the garden.

balance. It's fine to go wild from time to time, but an erratic lifestyle may play havoc with your cycles.

Seek herbal help. *Agnus castus* is an important herbal remedy for pre-menstrual syndrome, period pains, irregular cycles and hormone-related acne. It appears to exert a normalising influence on the pituitary gland and is best taken first thing in the morning when the pituitary is most active.

Chinese Angelica (*Angelica sinensis*) is a good tonic for women and helps to normalise oestrogen levels. It may ease menstrual cramps and reduce heavy bleeding. An infusion of lady's mantle can help relieve period pains. Sip three cups a day.

Use essential oils. Rose, geranium, cypress and nutmeg essential oils have a special affinity with the reproductive system and can help to normalise and restore menstrual cycles. Add 2–3 drops of your favourite essence to a teaspoon of carrier oil and massage into your tummy and lower back. Dissolve 10 drops in a tablespoon of organic milk for a rebalancing bath.

Seek out phyto-oestrogens. The beauty of plant oestrogens lies in their ability to buffer the effects of excessive oestrogen. This can help restore hormone balance and alleviate symptoms such as bloating, cravings for sweets, and may even help to prevent cellulite settling on the hips and thighs. Aim to include foods such as soya, chickpeas, lentils and mung beans which will provide the full spectrum of isoflavones in your diet.

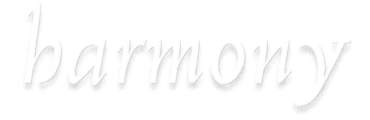

Pregnant Pause

In pregnancy, menstrual cycles are put on hold and a completely
different hormonal profile emerges.

This inevitably influences the skin's behaviour and appearance. The changes begin with a surge of human chorionic gonadotrophin hormone (HCG) secreted by the fertilised egg once it has settled in the womb. This hormone tells the corpus luteum (the empty follicle in the ovary) to keep making progesterone and stops the secretion of follicle stimulating hormone (responsible for starting another cycle). HCG seems responsible for the symptoms of morning sickness, but only in women who are especially sensitive to this hormone. When coupled with waves of fatigue characteristic of early pregnancy, skin can be left looking pale and lacking vitality.

NATURAL BLOOM

At around 12 weeks everything changes as the placenta takes charge of the hormonal situation. As well as allowing blood to flow between mother and baby, the placenta acts as a temporary endocrine organ. It secretes progesterone, oestrogen, HCG and human placental lactogen – the latter stimulates glands in the breasts to produce milk.

From the twelfth week onwards, progesterone levels steadily rise and skin enjoys a radiance unique to pregnancy. Make the most of this natural beauty by eating skin-nourishing foods, taking lots of gentle exercise (swimming, walking, yoga) and getting plenty of refreshing rest. Keeping the muscles firm throughout pregnancy will prevent loss of skin tone after the birth.

Just before the birth (at around 40 weeks), levels of progesterone fall and the pituitary starts producing oxytocin. This hormone stimulates uterine contractions and will initiate labour. Birth experiences vary enormously. If everything runs smoothly the body may produce lots of

IMPORTANT NOTE

It is not advisable to take herbal remedies during pregnancy (culinary herbs are fine, however). Many essential oils are unsafe to use, especially during the early months, but there are a few exceptions. These include rose, camomile, geranium, jasmine, sandalwood and ylang ylang, but do use them sparingly.

endorphins, natural painkillers which create feelings of euphoria and make the skin glow. Birth can also be intensely stressful and surges of adrenaline may leave skin looking pale and drained.

Looking after a tiny baby is always demanding. Sleepless nights and breast-feeding can sap the body's energy reserves and skin can reflect this fatigue. At this time it is essential to take extra care of yourself. Try a home-made spa treatment (see Chapters 5 and 6).

Tender loving care

Pregnancy may give your skin a new lease of life, but the changes at this time can be depleting, so treat yourself to some tender loving care.

Eat for two. While a growing baby increases your calorie needs by just 10 per cent, the optimum intake for certain nutrients during pregnancy can double. The recommended dose of folic acid rockets from around 400 to 800mcg a day during pregnancy. Other important pregnancy nutrients are calcium, zinc, iron, B vitamins, vitamin C and essential fatty acids, which are also essential for healthy skin. In early pregnancy your appetite may decline. Freshly made soups and juices are nourishing and slip down easily.

Keep supple. Skin is stretched and pulled as the baby grows. This can leave silvery-looking stretch marks on the thighs and tummy unless you take steps to keep skin ultra supple. Daily massage with a nutrient-rich oil is very good at preventing stretch marks. Zinc, vitamin C and silica are needed to keep and re-build strong, healthy collagen, so be sure you eat foods rich in these nutrients.

Take care of your breasts. As breasts get fuller during pregnancy and with breast-feeding, the skin here also gets stretched so be sure to keep it supple. Add 6 drops of rose essential oil to the Supple Skin Oil (page 122) and massage daily. After the baby is born, breasts can be prone to sagging, especially if you are breast-feeding. It is worth taking steps to restore firmness and tone (see page 93) as soon as possible.

Try touch treatment. Fluid retention is a common problem during the latter stages of pregnancy. To reduce swelling, drink plenty of pure spring water, and spend at least ten minutes a day lying down with a pillow under your feet. Manual lymphatic drainage is one of the best treatments for preventing and relieving this problem (see page 89).

The Cycle Ends

Like puberty, the menopause is a time of hormonal flux, but the
menstrual cycles are slowly winding down rather than starting up.

Women are born with hundreds of thousands of follicles in their ovaries. Over the years eggs mature within these follicles and are released with every passing cycle. Eventually there are too few follicles left for cycles to continue. Menopause is defined as having no periods for 12 months.

The average age for menopause is about 50, but many women begin experiencing hormonal changes that signal the onset of menopause in their forties or even late thirties. This early stage, often referred to as the peri-menopause, is remi-niscent of puberty. There may be skipped periods and, even during a regular cycle, ovulation may not occur which means progesterone levels fall. Progesterone has a very positive influence on the skin's texture and appearance, as we know from pregnancy, so this is bad news for skin.

FINAL FLING

During the peri-menopause, oestrogen seems to dominates the scene and this hormone imbal-ance triggers symptoms similar to pre-menstrual ones. They include feelings of anxiety, tearful-ness and irritability, as well as a tendency to fluid retention, headaches, poor digestion and even stomach cramps.

Because the ovaries respond spasmodically to follicle stimulating hormone (FSH) and luteiniz-ing hormone (LH), the pituitary pumps up increasing amounts to goad them into action. High levels of FSH and LH hormones seem responsible for hot flushes that make skin feel clammy.

When cycles eventually cease, oestrogen levels fall too. When this happens skin becomes

---

— Recipe —

SUPPLE SKIN OIL

30ml (2 tablespoons) sweet almond oil
15ml (1 tablespoon) wheatgerm oil
10 drops borage seed oil
10 drops carrot oil

Blend the oils together, store in a dark glass bottle and massage into the skin morning and evening. Keeps fresh for up to 6 months.

---

drier and thinner which encourages fine lines. The tiny capillaries that nourish skin become fragile and visible beneath the surface. Such changes are similar to those of ageing. While the hormonal upheavals of menopause are a part of life, there are lots of natural ways to make the transition easier.

FABULOUS PHYTOHORMONES – NATURE'S HRT

It has long been known that plants contain substances similar to human hormones. However, in the last decade research into these phytohormones has accelerated and findings so far hold enormous potential for women's health and beauty.

Plant hormones come into their own around the time of menopause because of their ability to buffer hormonal fluctuations. This makes the transition smoother and less disruptive. They also seem to supplement the body's own falling oestrogen and progesterone levels and so help to keep the skin looking younger for longer.

Know your phyto-oestrogens

Virtually every plant and plant food contains oestrogenic compounds. They belong to the broader family of flavonoids, plant substances with a phenolic structure similar to that of natu-

FOODS RICH IN PHYTO-OESTROGENS

alfalfa and bean sprouts	garlic	rye
	hops	sage
asparagus	legumes	sea vegetables
barley	liquorice	soya (as milk, tofu
celery	olive oil	and miso)
dates	onions	squash
fennel	papaya	sunflower seeds
figs	pears	wheatgerm
flax seeds	pomegranate	

rally produced oestrogens. This enables them to fit into oestrogen receptors. Although phyto-oestrogens are weaker than naturally produced oestrogens, they none the less seem to have a balancing influence within the body. They reduce the effects of excessive oestrogen and supplement falling levels. Studies suggest that women living in the Far East and Asia who eat lots of phyto-oestrogen-rich foods sail through the menopause with ease. They suffer fewer, if any, hot flushes and emotional problems. Their bones stay stronger and they are less at risk of suffering from heart disease. These hormone-enhancing benefits are also good news for the skin which ages faster when oestrogen levels fall.

The main families of phyto-oestrogens are:

Isoflavones ~ These are the most researched of

Gentle transition

๑ Keep your cool. Black cohosh, a herb traditionally known as 'squaw root' by Native Americans, may help reduce hot flushes. It is rich in phyto-oestrogens which seem to soothe the hypothalamus and reduce the pituitary's output of FSH and LH. *Agnus castus* has a similar influence on the hypothalamus, making it helpful during the menopause.

To stay cool and composed it helps to wear pure cotton clothes which allow the skin to breathe and to keep make-up as light as possible.

๑ Try skin supplements. As herbs like sage, hops and liquorice are oestreogenic, use them as frequently as possible. Try sipping infusions of sage or steeping sprigs of this herb in olive oil for salad dressings and using the leaves in cooking.

To help alleviate menopausal symptoms add about 2–3 drops of sage essential oil to a teaspoon of soya oil and massage into the skin.

๑ Be revived by rose. The most feminine of flowers, rose is a wonderful tonic for women and is particularly beneficial at this time of change. Sip infusions of rose petals, add rose essential oil to your bath and include it in skincare preparations.

๑ Build inner strength. Plant chemicals known as bioflavonoids help to strengthen and protect the blood capillaries from becoming fragile and easily damaged. They are present in the pith of citrus fruits such as lemon and grapefruit, and in red/blue berries such as strawberries, cherries, blueberries, raspberries and bilberries.

๑ De-sensitise. As the nervous system is already hyper-sensitive avoid anything that will aggravate it further. In place of stimulants like coffee and strong tea try drinking green tea and herbal tisanes. Yoga is excellent for relaxing the mind and body while certain postures are reputed to tone the pituitary and so balance hormonal secretions.

all phyto-oestrogens. There are four main types of isoflavone: genistein, diadzein, biochanin and formononetin. Different foods contain varying amounts of these isoflavones, but the richest sources are soya beans (including soya milk, soya sauce and tofu), chickpeas, lentils and mung beans.

🍃 Ideally try to eat some of these foods each day. All four isoflavones are found in red clover, a highly prized Native American herb. It can be taken as an infusion or in supplement form.

Lignans ~ These phytonutrients, like isoflavones, appear to regulate the body's oestrogen levels. Flax seeds (or linseeds) contain up to 800 times more lignans than most other plant foods.

🍃 Try adding a tablespoon of ground seeds to cereals and shakes, and use flax seed oil in salad dressings.

Replenishing progesterone

At present we know more about phyto-oestrogens than phytoprogesterones. The Mexican wild yam plant is the best-known natural source of a progesterone-like substance called diosgenin. From this compound, nature-identical progesterone is easily made. This is the active ingredient in natural progesterone creams and appears to be readily absorbed into the skin. Ordinary yams also appear to possess mild progestogenic qualities. Boiled, fried or roasted, they are popular in West African and Caribbean dishes.

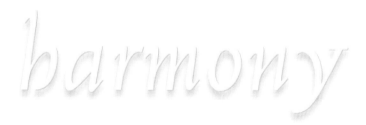

youthful

CHAPTER NINE

Age Control

~

The Essence of Youthfulness

Ageing is inevitable. From the moment we are born our biological clock starts to tick. But how well our skin weathers the passage of time is another story. Many things from the sun and stress to pollution and lack of exercise accelerate the ageing process. Anti-wrinkle creams may be helpful but they only skim the surface. The path to longer-lasting youth involves avoiding the things that make us age before our time and harnessing the help of skin-protective nutrients and regenerating plants. Knowing the ways of ageing holds the key to pre-serving skin's youthfulness, so wise up.

Be rejuvenated.

The Nature of Ageing

We live in a society that glorifies youth.

Most women wish their skin (and bodies) could look young forever. If there were an anti-wrinkle cream that really reversed the ageing process, it would be worth its weight in gold.

Not so long ago, ageing was believed to be entirely pre-programmed. We still tend to assume that wrinkles will appear when we hit 30 and from then on our skin's looks will slowly slide downhill. But nothing, it seems, is set in stone. Ageing is a complex affair. In the last 20 years we have started to question why it is that some people seem to age much more slowly than others. We now know for certain that sun exposure hastens the appearance of wrinkles. But skin also reflects what is happening within, and how young or old we look and feel is also influenced by all kinds of other factors. To look as young as possible, it is essential to tackle ageing from every angle.

VISIBLE SIGNS

The outward signs of ageing are all too familiar. First come very fine lines that are barely perceptible to the human eye. In the early days a moisturiser can smooth these away, for they are primarily due to lack of moisture in the superficial epidermal layers. This is partly because the sebaceous glands become less active as we get older. Oily skins have the advantage of being less vulnerable to fine lines.

As time passes the fine lines become permanently etched on the skin. This happens because of changes taking place deeper down in the skin's dermis. In this layer, collagen and elastin fibres are woven together to form a soft, springy mattress for the skin. In young-looking skin the fibres are arranged in neat orderly rows. Wrinkles and sagging occur when these fibres become bunched up and bonds known as cross-links form between them. This means the tissue becomes stiff and inelastic. As collagen binds and lends support to muscles, nerves, blood cells and organs throughout the body, everything becomes stiffer and less supple as we get older.

The speed of cell turnover also influences the skin's youthful looks although this process is invisible to the naked eye. In babies a new skin is being created every seven days because epidermal cells are dividing and moving to the surface so swiftly. The process slows down as we get older and by the time we are 70 it takes six weeks to create a new skin. Certain substances such as alpha-hydroxy acids (AHAs) applied to the skin can revv-up cell turnover, but their effects are only temporary.

So what does control the ageing process and to what extent can we influence it? The truth is that no one knows for certain, but scientists are coming closer than ever to unravelling the mysteries of ageing.

ALL IN THE GENES?

There is no doubt that genetics play a role in determining both the speed of ageing and longevity. It seems a biological clock encoded in our genetic material starts ticking the moment we are conceived and determines how long cells can live. Scientists have identified stretches of DNA (genetic material) known as telomeres at the ends of our genes. Each time a cell divides the telomere gets a little shorter. Cells seem to know how old they are because they can count the number of divisions they have made. When the telemere reaches a critical length, the cell is no longer able to divide. When this happens the damaged tissue cannot regenerate itself and dies. This is intrinsic ageing and there is little we can do about it. By tinkering with the genes scientists hope to control this process in the future.

Bio-technology has already tripled the lifespan of human skin cells.

There are also genes that are specifically concerned with ageing. Scientists have already found at least three and believe there are several hundred more. As genes are inherited, it explains why flawless skin tends to run in families.

MAKING MISTAKES

The gene theory explains why ageing is inevitable, but it is only part of the story. In fact some experts believe only about 25 per cent of ageing is genetic. The other 75 per cent has to be explained in other ways.

Another theory proposes that age-related changes are caused by the slow and gradual accumulation of errors. Our cells are constantly dividing and producing new cells. When cells reproduce themselves, their DNA must make an exact and perfect replica of itself. This does not always happen. Small errors may creep in when the DNA is being copied and these flaws are passed on to each new generation of cells. These errors give rise to defective enzymes and cell structures. They seem largely responsible for the changes that take place within the dermis that give rise to wrinkles. Mistakes occur naturally, but they can also be triggered by chemical entities known as free radicals. Controlling free-radical damage may be our best chance for holding back the ageing process.

Enemy within

Unlikely as it sounds, free radicals are derived from life-enhancing substances such as water and oxygen present in our bodily tissues. Free radicals are formed when molecules such as these are split into unstable and highly volatile fragments. Each molecule of oxygen, for example, is made from two atoms, hence the reason it is called O_2. When the molecule is split, the atoms separate and form singlet oxygen radicals or *Os. The * denotes a single electron (negatively charged particle) common to all free radicals. As electrons are more stable in pairs, a free radical will try to poach another electron from somewhere else.

Any of the cell's molecules seem fair game. When a free radical steals an electron from another molecule it generates yet another free radical and so a destructive chain reaction is set in motion. Free radicals move at the speed of

light and their chemical reactions take just a few millionths of a second. They are impossible to see or measure, but they leave a trail of destructive evidence in their wake. This is also known as oxidation damage.

Trail of destruction

Free radicals may attack fatty molecules in the cell membranes leaving them leaky and ineffective. As a result moisture seeps from the skin, leaving it dry and prone to fine lines. These disruptive entities may also penetrate the heart of the cell and alter its DNA, adding to the errors that occur naturally.

On a grand scale, free-radical damage leads to the gradual deterioration of tissues. As far as our skin is concerned it results in loss of smoothness, suppleness and the premature appearance of wrinkles. Some researchers go so far as to say that long-term free-radical damage not only accelerates ageing, but also plays a key role in the development of certain types of disease such as cancer.

> – Tip –
>
> Nip free radicals in the bud. Eat fresh fruit and a large leafy salad every day

Radical Thinking

With each breath, small quantities of oxygen get split into free radicals.
Is this inevitable or can we do something about it?

We know some things encourage free radicals to form. They are generated, for instance, when food and other substances are burned. Every puff of smoke produces thousands of free radicals. This explains why smoking results in the early appearance of wrinkles and can make the skin look ten years older than it is. Car exhaust fumes and chemical pollutants may also provoke the formation of free radicals.

Radiation is one of the worst offenders and includes the ultraviolet (UV) rays present in natural sunlight. UV rays are essentially packets of energy. When they strike the skin the sudden energy surge enables electrons to hop out of water and oxygen molecules, giving rise to hydroxy and singlet oxygen radicals.

Now here's the good news. We are blessed with an amazing free-radical defence system made up of antioxidant enzymes designed to stop these harmful substances in their tracks. What's more, evidence suggests that antioxidant nutrients present in a variety of foods play a key role in maintaining and supporting this fighting force.

– Reduce the radicals –

- Avoid alcohol.

- Stay away from smoky atmospheres.

- Don't eat burned, smoked, barbecued or fried food.

- Keep your windows up in polluted areas and escape from the city when you can.

- Opt for organic foods to avoid pesticides and other chemical residues on foods.

- Drink pure spring or mineral water – that on tap may contain oxidising nitrates and nitrites.

- Viral and bacterial infections generate free radicals (they may account for why we feel so groggy). Boost your antioxidant intake at these times.

- Don't over-expose yourself to strong sunlight.

NATURAL DEFENCES

Nature is clever. Our bodies are equipped with a whole army of enzymes capable of mopping up free radicals and limiting their damage potential. These age defenders are known as antioxidant

ANTIOXIDANT NUTRIENTS

Vitamin A and beta-carotene – These are important antioxidants that help to protect the cell membranes from free-radical attacks.

- Good sources include fish oils, carrots, apricots, cantaloupe melon, green leafy vegetables.

Vitamin C – One of nature's potent antioxidants. As well as mopping up free radicals itself, vitamin C recharges vitamin E and glutathione (a substance present inside cells which deals with free radicals that slip past vitamin E). As vitamin C is water-soluble it cannot be stored in the tissues and must be replenished on a daily basis.

- Good sources include citrus fruits, green peppers, broccoli, Brussels sprouts, blackcurrants, redcurrants, mango, kiwi fruit, papaya, cantaloupe melon.

Vitamin E – This nestles in the cell membranes and snags any free radical that comes along, so protecting the fatty acids in the membranes from oxidation.

- Good sources include dried apricots, mango, olive oil, assorted nuts, pumpkin and sunflower seeds, wheat-germ, sweet potato, kale.

Copper – Found in soya beans, legumes, whole wheat, prunes, liver, seafood, molasses.

Manganese – This is present in leafy green vegetables, wholegrains, tea.

Selenium – This is present in fish such as salmon, mackerel and tuna as well as nuts (especially brazil nuts), seeds.

Zinc – Found in oysters, shellfish, chicken, sunflower and pumpkin seeds, assorted nuts, legumes, peas.

enzymes and each seems to be specially designed to deal with a particular brand of free radical. They include superoxide dismutase (SOD) – which soaks up the superoxide radical – catalase and glutathione perioxidase.

These enzymes rely on certain nutrients such as the minerals selenium, zinc, manganese and copper to work efficiently. Like all enzymes they become less effective as we age and so our natural protection from free radicals declines with the passing years.

Luckily certain vitamins act as antioxidants in their own right and keeping levels well topped up may be one of the best ways to keep wrinkles at bay.

Skin and the Sun

There is no question that soaking up the sun's rays encourages the early formation of wrinkles.

Some dermatologists go so far as to say that 80–90 per cent of wrinkles are sun induced.

If sun exposure were kept to a bare minimum, our skin might be free from wrinkles and age spots into our eighties. This may be true, but on the flip side of the coin skin almost always looks healthier for a dose of fresh air and sunshine. Being in the sun also has far-reaching psychological benefits. Feeling relaxed, happy and good about ourselves shines from within. It is easy to understand how lying out on a beach all day long in the blazing Mediterranean sun can wreak havoc on skin, but in between charcoal-grilled and pasty white lies healthy balance.

For your skin's sake, give up sunbathing. Sacrifice the deep bronzed look for a light, golden sun-kissed glow that can be achieved by minimal exposure. At the same time maximise antioxidant protection to prevent free radicals from doing their worst.

SUN FACTS

Sunlight contains UVA, UVB and UVC rays. All the UVC is deflected back into outer space by the earth's atmospheric shield. So, by the time sunlight reaches our skin it is composed of all the colours of the visible light spectrum, plus UVB and UVA rays. There are the short wave infrared, micro- and radio-waves at one end of the spectrum and longer ultraviolet (UV) rays at the other. The ultraviolet rays fall into two factions. The UVB rays (wavelength 280 to 320 nanometres (nm)) are the so-called burning rays. They penetrate the upper layers of the epidermis and the damage they do is obvious. After excessive exposure to UVB, skin becomes pink and inflamed.

The longer UVA rays (wavelength 320 to 400nm) sink deeper into the skin and reach the dermis. The damage they do to the collagen and elastin fibres is not immediately visible and reveals itself several years later as lines and wrinkles.

The proportion of UV radiation in sunlight varies according to the time of day (peaking around midday), season, altitude and location.

In the UK around 130 times the amount of UV radiation reaches the skin at noon in mid-summer as opposed to mid-winter. The closer we move to the equator, the greater the proportion of UV rays present in sunlight. However, thinning of the ozone layer in the northern hemisphere may change all that. Ozone filters all of the sun's most harmful UVC plus some UVB and A. In recent years the summer sun in northern climes appears to have increased its burning potential.

IN-BUILT SUNSHADE

A tan is simply the skin's way of defending itself from the sun. When UV light falls on the skin, cells lying at the base of the epidermis known as melanocytes leap into action and start making a brown pigment known as melanin. The cells have long spindly arms and they squirt melanin into neighbouring cells. This pigment then forms a natural sunshade over the nucleus (which contains the cell's DNA) to shield it from incoming UV rays.

Melanin is powerful stuff. As well as absorbing and reflecting UV rays, it also does a wonderful job of mopping up free radicals.

As the cells rise to the surface, the layer of pigment moves upwards and is eventually shed along with the horny cells of the stratum corneum.

Melanin provides the skin with a natural and in-built sun protection factor (SPF) of anything from 2 up to 9. So if we are going to be in the sun it would seem a distinct advantage to have an even and protective tan.

But there are drawbacks. To begin with, cells are being damaged before the melanin provides an adequate shield. It takes about 48 hours for colour to appear, during which time the skin is particularly vulnerable.

Although we all have exactly the same number of melanocytes, they vary in the quality, rate and quantity of melanin they produce. Your ability to tan is genetic. Some people with very fair Celtic complexions only produce the pale, reddish-brown variety, phaeomelanin, which offers very poor sun protection. Deep brown eumelanin is far more protective and may afford skin a much higher SPF. Skin type is inherited and it is important to know how well your skin can rally its defences against the sun's rays. By its very nature fair skin will always be more vulnerable to sun-induced ageing than those of olive tones.

What is an SPF?

Different skin types burn more easily than others. For very pale, freckly skin just five minutes exposure to sunlight can cause erythema (sunburn). The minimum amount of sun

KNOW YOUR SKIN TYPE

SKIN TYPE	IN THE SUN	EXTRA PROTECTION
1 very fair, often freckled, blonde or red hair	always burns, never tans, natural SPF 1	SPF 25–30
2 fair skin, blonde, blue/green eyes	burns readily, tans but slowly, natural SPF 1.5	SPF 15–20
3 medium skin tone, light brown hair	burns at first, then turns golden brown, natural SPF 2.5	SPF 15
4 olive skin, brown eyes, Mediterranean type	rarely burns, tans easily, natural SPF 4	SPF 8–15
5 dark Far Eastern, Indian	hardly ever burns, tans deeply, natural SPF 6.5	SPF 8
6 black African, Caribbean	never burns, colour darkens, natural SPF 9	SPF 6

exposure to cause sunburn is known as minimal erythemal dose (MED). Most fair skins can tolerate up to 15 minutes of sun exposure before their skin starts to turn pink. The sun protection factor extends the time you can spend in the sun before burning. An SPF of 2 means you can stay out in the sun for 2 x 15 minutes, while an SPF of 10 extends this time to 150 minutes.

That's in theory. In real terms creams get rubbed off and washed away. Top up the protection every hour with a thick layer of cream – at least 1 teaspoon's worth for your face alone.

Protective Preparations

The burning power of the sun varies during the day, reaching a peak
at around midday, so it is advisable to stay out of the sun between
11am and 3pm.

People who live in hot countries always stay in the shade during the middle of the day.

If you must venture out in the sun when the UV rays are most potentially damaging, it is essential to boost your sun protection factor irrespective of whether your skin is lightly tanned or not.

WHAT'S IN A SUNSCREEN?

Physical blocks ~ These creams rely on micro-reflective particles, usually of titanium dioxide, to deflect and reflect the sun's UV rays away from the skin. They are usually opaque and form an occlusive film on the skin. They are effective and well tolerated.

Chemical blocks ~ These preparations may be gels, mousses and creams. They contain chemicals capable of absorbing UV rays, rather like melanin itself. In doing so, their structure changes and they reach a saturation point which means they have to be reapplied every hour or less. The combination of chemicals, UV light and heat means these sunscreens easily irritate sensitive skins.

Antioxidants ~ Flooding the skin cells with antioxidant nutrients such as beta-carotene, vitamin E and C may help to mop up free radicals as they are formed, so preventing them from causing damage. These nutrients may boost the skin's natural SPF by a factor of 2. For the best effects they should be applied before, during and after sun exposure.

SUN PROTECTION FROM WITHIN

Flooding your skin with antioxidants from without and within may be an effective way to boost its natural sun protection factor. In addition to antioxidant nutrients such as vitamins A, C and E, research reveals that there is a vast array of antioxidant compounds in plants. Some of these seem to have a special affinity with the skin and are often far more potent than other antioxidants. They may help to neutralise the sudden surge of free radicals that occurs when skin is exposed to UV rays. To maximise skin protection, ensure your diet contains plenty of these phytonutrients throughout the summer months.

Carotenoids ~ There are around 20 or so different carotenoids in fruits and vegetables, the best known being beta-carotene (which we convert to vitamin A). Their role in plants is to offer protection from UV damage and they may do the same for us, too. We know carotenoids in foods reach the skin because eating too many carrots gives it an orange hue. When present at the skin's surface they appear to absorb and scatter sunlight so it cannot penetrate the deeper layers. They also seem to soak up free radicals. Research shows that supplementing the diet with 50mg of mixed carotenoids for five weeks provides fair-skinned people with a natural SPF of between 2 and 4.

Carotenoids include, in order of potency:

- Lycopene, bright red, present in tomatoes.
- Lutein and zeaxanthin, yellowish, present in spinach and kale.
- Alpha-carotene, orange, present in pumpkins and carrots.

- Cryptoxanthin, orange, present in papayas, mangoes and tangerines.
- Beta-carotene, orange, but may be overshadowed by the green pigment chlorophyll in plants. Present in broccoli, carrots, sweet potatoes, yellow squash, spinach, tomatoes, kale, cantaloupe melons.

Alpha-lipoic acid ~ One of the most recently discovered natural antioxidants. Initial findings suggest this substance may slow down UV-related ageing and it is being added to a new generation of wrinkle creams. Present in spinach.

Anthocyanidins ~ These are flavonoid compounds with powerful antioxidant properties found in purple and blue fruits. The free-radical quenching potency of the oligomeric proanthocyanidin complex (in black grapes and red wine) is thought to be 20 times stronger than vitamin C. This complex also has anti-inflammatory properties that may help to soothe sunburn. Anthocyanidins and proanthocyanidins are also stronger than vitamin E. Present in black grapes, blueberries, blackcurrants, strawberries, raspberries, cherries, cranberries, bilberries.

— Recipe —
ANTIOXIDANT SERUM

This serum is rich in antioxidant nutrients and provides a mild SPF of around 2 which helps to nip free-radical damage in the bud. Apply before and after sun exposure. Sinks swiftly into the skin and can be worn under your moisturiser or sunscreen.

1 teaspoon of green tea or a tea bag
300ml (1 pint) just-boiled pure spring water
2 teaspoons freshly squeezed lemon juice
1 tablespoon aloe vera gel
20 drops carrot oil
1 capsule vitamin E oil
6 drops orange essential oil

Infuse the green tea in steaming hot spring water for 10–15 minutes. Remove the tea bag or strain the tea leaves away and add the lemon juice. Spoon the aloe vera gel into a small glass bowl, add the carrot oil and squeeze the vitamin E oil from the capsule. Stir these together and then add 2 tablespoons of the green tea and lemon mix when cool. Finally add the orange essential oil and decant into a small, tinted glass bottle, preferably with a pump dispenser and shake well. Use about half a teaspoonful for the face. Keeps fresh for up to 1 week when chilled.

SAFE IN THE SUN

- Always protect pale skin from the sun.

- Never exceed the MED (i.e. don't let your skin turn pink).

- Even if your skin is tanned, always supplement its natural SPF in strong sunlight.

- Stay out of the midday sun during the summer months and in hot countries. The safest time to be in the sun is before 11am and after 3pm.

- Never rely on a sunscreen alone for all-day protection.

- Before and after sun exposure saturate your skin with natural antioxidants.

- Remember that the sun's rays penetrate water, so if you go swimming wear a T-shirt or a waterproof sunscreen.

- The higher the altitude the greater the proportion of UVB in the sun's rays. When skiing always go for high-level sun protection. The rays are reflected off snow and ice making them even more lethal.

Sunproof Diet

During the summer months it makes sense to include as many
antioxidant-rich foods into your diet as possible.
Here are some suggestions.

❧ Breakfast – stir fresh strawberries, raspberries, blueberries or cherries into natural live yoghurt.

Soak dried apricots, peaches and prunes in pure spring water overnight, then strain and sprinkle with flaked almonds.

❧ Snacks – peaches, raisins, carrots, fresh cherries, sunflower and pumpkin seeds.

❧ Lunch and Dinner – make a cool gazpacho soup with fresh tomatoes, red and green peppers, onion and cucumber with lemon juice.

Serve pasta with a sauce made from tomatoes, onion, garlic and basil.

Eat a green salad which includes young spinach leaves, broccoli florets and green peppers every day.

Make a Greek salad with tomatoes, red and green peppers, cucumber and onion.

❧ Dessert – serve fresh papaya with lime juice.

Make a fresh fruit salad of cantaloupe melon, mango and red grapes.

Lightly stew a mixture of summer fruits such as strawberries, redcurrants, blackcurrants, raspberries, blackberries and blueberries.

❧ Drinks – sip fresh carrot, mango and orange juices.

Whizz up fresh strawberry and raspberry milkshakes and sprinkle with wheatgerm for extra vitamin E.

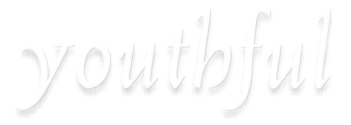

Young as You Feel

Protecting skin from environmentally induced ageing
is one way to preserve its youthful looks. But skin reflects
what is going on inside too.

It is becoming clear that there are two sorts of ageing. Chronological or time-linked ageing relates to changes that occur with time. It has always been the yardstick by which we measure youth and its gradual demise. However, there is another kind of ageing which also influences just how young or old we feel and look.

Biological ageing is not bound to time. It is more to do with how well cells are renewing themselves and how efficiently they are using oxygen. Unlike chronological age, your biological age can be changed – for better or worse. You can be young and have a high biological age, or in your middle years and have a biological age of someone in their twenties.

Biological age is essentially a measure of inner vitality and energy. The higher your vitality levels, the lower your biological age.

By the age of 35 we are beginning to lose cells in our brain and other vital organs including the heart and skin, so those left behind have to work harder and use ever greater amounts of energy.

This explains why energy levels decline with age.

Some people seem blessed with more vitality than others. But there are ways to enhance your vitality and so reduce your biological age. When you feel younger, you also look younger and skin is no exception.

TURN BACK TIME

Be active. Activity works wonders for knocking years off your biological age because it helps the body to use oxygen more efficiently. All the things that get worse as you get older (lung capacity, circulation, cardiovascular fitness) improve when you exercise. The more active you are, the greater your energy and vitality levels. Research shows that 40 minutes of daily exercise adds 12 years to your life. If you want to look five to eight years younger than you really are in middle life take three brisk one-mile (1·6 km) walks a week.

Chill out. Stress accelerates the ageing process. Deep wrinkles or worry lines are just that – they reflect our inner stress. In youth, emotions flit momentarily across our faces, but over the years deep muscle tension and loss of elasticity mean our emotions become indelibly etched in our skin. At this stage it may take more than daily relaxation or a refreshing holiday to shift some of those lines. What you need is a complete emotional detox. It is time to re-evaluate your life. This may involve ditching relationships which make you feel angry and frustrated, and seeing things in a different perspective. Discovering inner happiness and a sense of fulfilment will knock years off your life and your skin.

Make a face. Exercising the muscles of the face, as well as the body, is a good way to prevent skin from sagging, especially around the jawline. Specific face work-outs can give the face a natural lift and take years off your appearance. Typical exercises include grimacing, opening the mouth wide and closing it again, raising and relaxing the eyebrows.

Eat antioxidant food. A diet rich in antioxidants really can help to slow down the ageing process in the body. As many fruits and vegeta-bles contain a variety of different antioxidants from vitamins C and E to carotenoids and flavonoids, a team of researchers at the Human Research Centre on Ageing at Tuft's University in America set out to test their total ability to soak up oxygen-derived free radicals. They measured their oxygen radical absorbency power and found that prunes came top of the list. A 100g (3½oz) serving raised the antioxidant power of blood by 25 per cent.

If you want to stay young for longer, be sure to eat some of the foods listed below each day.

Spring-clean your body. Detoxing is a great way to boost vitality and rejuvenate your body. If you want to stay young it is a good idea to have a thorough spring-clean whenever you feel tired and your skin looks drab. Try to detox for

TOP ANTIOXIDANT FRUITS AND VEGETABLES

(in order of free radical absorbing power)

1. prunes	7. plums	13. broccoli
2. raisins	8. oranges	14. beetroot
3. blueberries	9. black grapes	15. red peppers
4. blackberries	10. kale	16. onion
5. strawberries	11. spinach	17. sweetcorn
6. raspberries	12. Brussels sprouts	18. cherries

at least three days and preferably a week. Give up coffee and alcohol, eat nothing but fresh vegetables, fruits, wholegrains, live natural yoghurt, nuts, seeds and legumes on your detox. Drink masses of pure spring water and herbal infusions. Take hot and cold showers, body brush daily and take plenty of long walks in the fresh air.

Spice up your sex life. Research shows that people who seem much younger than their years have fulfilling relationships and satisfying sex lives. Sexual intercourse triggers the release of various beneficial chemicals, including small amounts of growth hormone, which reduce fatty

tissue and increase lean muscle giving skin a sleeker, more youthful appearance. Orgasm increases the blood flow to the skin and the secretion of endorphins, pleasure chemicals which make skin glow.

Stretch yourself. Our bodies become increasingly inflexible with age. As muscle tensions become entrenched and joints lose mobility, the blood flows less freely to the skin and other organs. Regular stretching is one of the best ways to preserve a lithe and supple physique. Try taking up a gentle form of yoga or pilates.

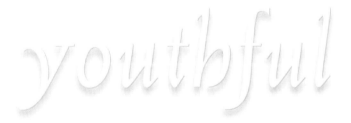

Nature's Rejuvenators

The search for an elixir of youth is centuries old.

The ancient Chinese emperors and Egyptian pharaohs thought it possible not just to preserve youth but ultimately to attain immortality. They turned to plants, herbs and flowers to help them achieve eternal youth. We now know ageing is our destiny, but science confirms that some of these old remedies might help to preserve youthful energy, vitality and looks.

FROM WITHIN

Ginseng ~ Traditionally used in Chinese medicine to ward off the effects of ageing. Ginseng is renowned for its ability to prolong endurance and vigour, qualities that dwindle in later life. This nourishing and strengthening herb helps to relieve tiredness and fatigue associated with ageing. It also has a reputation for revitalising the sex glands. The gradual decline of sex hormones that begins in the middle years seems partly responsible for symptoms of ageing.

TOP TEN
ANTI-AGEING
ESSENTIAL
OILS

frankincense

geranium

lavender

lemon

myrrh

neroli

patchouli

rose

rosemary

thyme

For best results avoid acid fruit juices such as orange, grapefruit and vitamin C for three hours after taking ginseng as they neutralise its beneficial effects.

Schisandra ~ A Tibetan medicine traditionally used to help preserve the adaptability of youth. In folklore, schisandra comes from Shangri-La, the legendary valley of everlasting youth and has been used for nearly 5,000 years. Travellers to Tibet have been struck by the advanced age of many locals who reputedly owe their youthful strength, energy and alertness to schisandra.

Ginkgo biloba (maidenhair tree) ~ Another Chinese herb prized for enhancing and extending life. This majestic tree has been in existence for over 200 million years and its species has survived giant meteor strikes, ice ages and rising pollution levels.

MINI FACELIFT

- Stroke both hands up the neck to the chin, then up and over the ears.
- Pinch the skin with the thumb and first finger and work along the jawline.
- Using the back of your hands alternately pat under the chin.
- Make scissoring movements across the forehead.
- Pinch the eyebrows.
- With the forefingers apply circular pressure to the temples.

Ginkgo contains some potent antioxidants, namely its unique flavonoid ginkgolides and quercetin. These strengthen and protect tiny blood capillaries while improving oxygen supply to the skin and other tissues.

FOR THE SKIN

Essential oils ~ These are anti-ageing because they promote cell renewal, a process which gradually slows down as we get older. Gentle stimulation of the sebaceous glands helps to keep the skin well-lubricated and moisturised. Massaged into the skin on a daily basis, essential oils can help to preserve smoothness and suppleness, as well as helping to reverse some early signs of degeneration. Frankincense is particularly renowned for its regenerating and rejuvenating properties.

Uplifting massage ~ Face wrinkles, unlike those in the rest of our body, are inserted into the skin. This means that massaging the skin is a wonderful way to release the tension that encourages deep frown and anxiety lines. Upward stroking movements also help to counter the effects of gravity, and massaging the face on a daily basis can provide a natural facelift.

To enhance the benefits, use the **Rejuvenating Massage Oil** opposite.

Wrinkle-smoothing herbs ~ Some herbs help to soften the skin and may also encourage cell regeneration, so they are good to include in anti-ageing creams and lotions. These include comfrey, elderflower, marshmallow, lime blossom, lady's mantle.

— Recipes —

REJUVENATING MASSAGE OIL

2 drops rose essential oil
2 drops geranium essential oil
1 drop patchouli essential oil
1 teaspoon apricot or peach kernel oil
1 teaspoon borage oil
1 teaspoon wheatgerm oil

Blend all the oils together and store in a small tinted glass bottle. Use in conjunction with facelift massage. Keeps fresh for up to 6 months.

INSTANT COOL SPRAY

To refresh skin when the temperature climbs, add 4 teaspoons of vegetable glycerine to your favourite floral water (see pages 22–3). Pour into a small spritzer bottle and spray.

WRINKLE SMOOTHING CREAM

1 teaspoon cocoa butter
1 teaspoon white beeswax
1 teaspoon emulsifying wax
1 tablespoon apricot or peach kernel oil
10 drops carrot oil
10 drops borage oil
2 tablespoons lime blossom or elderflower
   infusion
1 teaspoon vegetable glycerine
1 capsule vitamin E
2 drops rose essential oil
2 drops neroli essential oil
1 drop frankincense essential oil

Melt the cocoa butter, beeswax and emulsifying wax in a small glass bowl over a saucepan of simmering water. Slowly add in the apricot, carrot and borage oils, stirring with a wooden spoon until well blended, then stir in the herbal infusion and the vegetable glycerine. Remove from the heat and squeeze in the Vitamin E oil from the capsule. When cool, stir in the essential oils and spoon into a small jar. Keep cool and preferably chilled. Lasts for up to 4 weeks.

perfect

skin

CHAPTER TEN

28 Days
to
Perfect Skin

~

Every day new skin cells are being born. On average it takes around 28 days, a few less in your twenties and a few more as you get older, for these cells to travel up to the surface. This provides endless opportunities for improving your skin. This 28-day programme will show you how to draw upon all the essential skin-perfecting elements and weaves them together into a weekly maintenance regime for keeping your skin in tip-top condition. It takes just 28 days to re-create your skin, so begin today.

Be renewed.

Days 1–4
4 DAYS OF CLEANSING

DAY 1

Cleansing

Choose your perfect cleansing ritual (see page 15) based on your skin right now.

DAY 2

Exfoliating

For the face ~ After your morning cleanse, take a teaspoon of clear honey and smooth it over your skin. With the fingertips, pat quickly repeatedly all over the face for about 5 minutes. Rinse off with warm water and spray or dab with a refresher. In the evening, replace your normal cleansing milk or cream with a skin-polishing cream such as **Pineapple or Papaya Peel** (page 25) for dry and sensitive skins, or **Almond Refining Cream** (page 25) for normal or oily skins. Massage gently into the skin reaching into every corner, then whisk away with a damp muslin cloth. Spray with a floral refresher.

For the body ~ Before showering or bathing, rub a body exfoliating scrub like **Lavender and Almond Body Polisher** (page 25) into the skin using circular massage movements, concentrating on rough areas such as knees and elbows. Shower away with warm water or rinse off in the bath.

DAY 3

Steam cleaning

For the face ~ After your morning or evening cleansing ritual (whenever suits you best) do a steam-clean facial (page 25). To encourage deep cleansing, add a few drops of camomile or lavender essential oils or infuse with elderflower or yarrow.

For a cleansing boost, take a square of muslin or gauze (large enough to cover your face) and soak in wheatgrass juice. Gently squeeze out the excess then lay over the face like a compress and relax for 10 minutes. Finish by spraying or dabbing skin with a floral refresher.

For the body ~ Take a dry sauna or Turkish steam bath. For a cleansing boost or a home-spa alternative to steaming, pour and pat wheatgrass juice all over your skin at bathtime, allowing the excess to dissolve in the bathwater. Soak for 15–20 minutes, rinse with fresh water and wrap yourself in a warm towel.

DAY 4

Deep cleansing

For the face ~ Choose and prepare an appropriate clay-based mask for your skin. After your morning or evening cleansing ritual (whenever suits you best) apply to the face and neck area. Leave for 10–15 minutes before rinsing off and finish by spraying with a floral refresher.

For the body ~ Using specially prepared mud such as Italian 'fango' or Dead Sea mud, smear a thin layer all over the body and leave on for 15–20 minutes. Rinse off with warm water or,

better still, toss a handful of sea salt into a bath and soak for another 10–15 minutes.

Cleansing supplements

- Take 20 drops of echinacea tincture three times a day.
- Drink 25ml (1fl oz) wheatgrass or watercress juice neat or diluted with carrot or apple juice.
- Stir 1 teaspoon of psyllium husks into juice or sprinkle over breakfast cereal.
- Drink 2 cups of a specially formulated detox tea (for stockist see page 197).

Days 1–4: daily cleansing plan

As well as following the blueprint for healthy eating (page 51) focus on cleansing foods for the blood, lymph, liver, kidneys and large intestine.

- On rising, drink a cup of hot water and half the juice of a freshly squeezed lemon.
- Add berry fruits such as strawberries, raspberries and blueberries to a breakfast bowl of natural live yoghurt or muesli.
- Eat a large mixed green salad every day. Include lots of chlorophyll-rich vegetables such as spinach, lamb's lettuce, cos lettuce, endive, dandelion leaves and sprouted alfalfa.
- For a sustaining evening meal choose soup made from watercress, spinach, asparagus, artichoke, onion or beetroot. Season with parsley and garlic.
- Nibble on chunks of apple and pear, celery sticks and slices of pepper.
- Avoid drinking coffee and alcoholic drinks on these cleansing days. Sip peppermint and green tea, drink lots of pure spring water and freshly squeezed juices, especially apple, grapefruit and black grape.

Days 5–8

4 DAYS OF MOISTURISING AND RESTORING FLUID BALANCE

DAY 5

Begin by making or choosing a moisturiser such as **Rose Petal Moisturiser** (see page 38) to suit your skin, as well as a body lotion like **Jasmine Skin Drink** (see page 39).

Moisture boost

For the face ~ After cleansing and refreshing, make a moisture mask by soaking a piece of muslin or gauze in rose petal and marshmallow infusion, squeezing out the excess and placing over the face. Leave for 5–10 minutes, then apply your moisturiser.

For the body ~ Make a moisturising bath by placing a handful of rose petals or marshmallow root in a muslin bag. Hang from the tap so the water runs through it and then leave to steep in the bath. After drying, apply body lotion.

DAY 6

Water therapy

For the face ~ Decant some Evian or your

Days 5–8: *daily water-balancing plan*

- Drink a glass of water first thing each morning and last thing before going to sleep. Be sure to drink at least 1 litre (1³/₄ pints) of pure spring water throughout the day.
- Avoid any salty foods such as crisps, salted nuts, bacon, sausages and processed food of any kind.
- Eat plenty of fluid-balancing foods, especially watermelon, cucumber, celery and asparagus. Bananas are a good potassium-rich snack.
- Add baby dandelion leaves and endive to salads.
- Moisturise from within by enriching your diet with essential fatty acids. Combine equal quantities of sunflower, pumpkin, flax and sesame seeds (around 50g (2oz) of each) and place in a blender. Sprinkle your four-seed combo over breakfast cereal and soups. (Keep chilled in a sealed container to prevent the oils going rancid.)

favourite pure spring water into a spritzer bottle and spray your skin first thing in the morning, before applying your moisturiser, and frequently throughout the day.

For the body ~ Spray the body or take a shower alternating between hot and cold water. Begin with warm, then switch to cold for 30–60 seconds, then turn back to warm (see also page 42). Follow with body lotion.

DAY 7

Softening and replenishing

For the face ~ For an intensive softening treatment, mix together 1 teaspoon of aloe vera gel and 1 teaspoon of clear honey, plus 1 drop of rose or geranium essential oil, then smooth over the face. Leave for 10 minutes, then splash off with warm water. Pat dry and apply your moisturiser.

For the body ~ Spoon 1 tablespoon of oatmeal into a small muslin bag and hang on the bath tap so water runs through it, then place in the bath to steep. Add 3 drops of rose essence to your bath and soak for a good 15 minutes. Pat dry and moisturise.

— *Recipe* —
REPLENISHING OIL

1 tablespoon sweet almond oil
10 drops evening primrose or borage oil
1 teaspoon wheatgerm oil
3 drops geranium essential oil
3 drops sandalwood essential oil

Mix the oils together in a small glass bowl and then drop in the essential oils. Apply to the face and/or body. After 10–15 minutes tissue off the excess, spray the skin with a refresher and then moisturise.

DAY 8

Restoring skin's protective barrier

For the face and body ~ After your evening cleansing ritual and a warm bath or shower, massage the skin with the above oil blend.

Moisturising supplements

- Take 1 tablespoon of cold-pressed flax oil or an oil blend that provides equal quantities of omega 3 and 6 fatty acids daily. Use in salad dressings, drizzle over steamed vegetables or take in capsule form.

- Drink 2 cups of fennel or golden rod tea a day.

Days 9–12
4 DAYS OF NOURISHING AND REPLENISHING

DAY 9

Nutrient boost

For the face ~ After evening cleansing and refreshing, massage 1 teaspoon of a nutrient-rich fluid or serum like **Nourishing Serum** (see page 70) into your skin.

For the body ~ Buff your skin with a salty scrub (see page 45) made by blending a little sea salt with some olive oil, then soak for 15 minutes in a **Seaweed Bath** (see page 46) scented with a few drops of lavender essence. Shower off any seaweed residue, wrap up warmly in a towel and rest for a further 10–15 minutes.

DAY 10

Skin supplement

For the face ~ After morning or evening cleansing, prepare a nourishing mask – see **Skin Supplement**, page 70 – or simply whizz half an avocado in the blender with 1 teaspoon of honey and add 2 drops of orange essential oil. Apply after your usual morning or evening cleansing ritual and leave on the skin for 10 minutes before rinsing away with warm water. Refresh and mois-

turise. After evening cleansing, apply your **Nourishing Serum** (see page 70).

For the body ~ After a warm bath or shower, massage the skin with 1 tablespoon of avocado oil and 6 drops of orange essential oil.

DAY 11

Skin soak

For the face ~ As for day 9.

For the body ~ Add 2 tablespoons of powdered milk and 6 drops of a favourite essential oil to your bath. Soak for 15–20 minutes, shower with warm, then cold water before drying.

DAY 12

Intensive nourishment

For the face ~ After morning cleansing apply another nourishing mask. Try blending half a banana with 1 tablespoon of natural yoghurt and 1 teaspoon of wheatgerm oil or choose your favourite. Liquidise for a creamy consistency, apply a thick layer and leave for 10 minutes, then rinse away with warm water and pat dry. After

Days 9–12: daily nourishing plan

- Start the day with a nourishing smoothie drink. Just toss the recipe ingredients (below) into a blender.
- Eat a few slices of fresh pineapple or papaya after each meal to aid digestion.
- Work as many of the nourishing foods (see pages 64–5) into your daily diet as possible. Eat a selection of fresh vegetables with every meal. Have at least one green leafy salad made with a good handful of fresh watercress each day. Snack on carrot sticks, apples and pears.
- Sprinkle flaked seaweed into your stir-fries and soups.
- Carry a small bag of mixed almonds, hazelnuts, walnuts, sesame seeds, pumpkin seeds and sultanas with you. Nibble on these if you feel hungry between meals.

evening cleansing apply **Nourishing Serum** (see page 70).

For the body ~ Treat yourself to a **Seaweed Body Wrap** (see page 46).

Nourishing supplements

- Take 2 tablets of spirulina or chlorella twice a day, or a heaped teaspoon of green superfood supplement (for stockists see pages 197–9).
- Take a freeze-dried probiotic supplement morning and evening.

– Recipe –
BREAKFAST SMOOTHIE

2 tablespoons live natural yoghurt

150–200ml (5–7fl oz) organic milk or fresh juice

1 banana

115g (4oz) favourite fruit such as raspberries, strawberries, blueberrries, mango or peach

1 tablespoon four-seed mix

1 teaspoon rice or wheatgerm

Whizz together until creamy, pour into a long glass and sprinkle with cinnamon or nutmeg.

Days 13–16
4 DAYS OF DE-STRESSING AND RELAXATION

DAY 13

Stress relief

For the whole person

Turn to page 106 and select a flower remedy that best describes how you feel right this moment. Add a few drops to a glass of water or cup of herbal tea and drink first thing each morning.

Put a small amount of moisturiser in the palm of your hand, add 1 drop of flower remedy and blend them together before applying to your face. You can add 2 drops to your body lotion too.

Do this each morning for the next 3 days.

DAY 14

Soothing

For the face ~ After your morning or evening cleansing ritual, massage some **Soothing Massage Oil** (see page 105) into your face. Use very light, soothing strokes. With your forefinger apply circling pressure to the point between your eyebrows to work away tension. Tissue off the excess oil before refreshing and moisturising.

  Sometime during the day or evening practise a Mini meditation (see page 99). Scent the air with sandalwood or frankincense essential oil to create a calming atmosphere.

Days 13–16: daily de-stressing plan

- Begin the day with a breakfast based on oats (such as muesli or porridge) with chopped banana or fresh figs.
- If you feel agitated, nibble a few almonds during the day.
- Avoid stimulants like coffee and strong tea. Instead sip soothing camomile and elderflower tisanes. To aid a good night's sleep add a teaspoon of orange flower water to a cup of hot water and sweeten with honey.
- Aim to do 30 minutes of vigorous aerobic exercise each day to burn off any pent-up adrenaline.

DAY 15

Banishing tension

Head massage ~ Ideal to do just before washing your hair. Using the tips of all your fingers and thumbs, massage your scalp. Be quite firm and apply circling movements to release tension. Work down the neck with soothing strokes and out across the shoulder blades. Ideally get someone else to give you this massage treatment.

- In the evening relax in a long, soothing bath. Dissolve up to 10 drops of a tranquillising essential oil such as neroli or sandalwood in a tablespoon of organic milk before adding to the bathwater.

DAY 16

Dream away

For the face ~ A soothing massage as on day 14.

- Sometime during the day or evening practise a dream visualisation (see page 100). Scent the room with sandalwood or frankincense essential oils to create a calming atmosphere.

Soothing supplements

- Take 20 drops of kava kava tincture in water 3 times a day.

- Book yourself a full one-hour body massage.

- Do a 10–15 minute meditation each day (see Mini meditation, page 99).

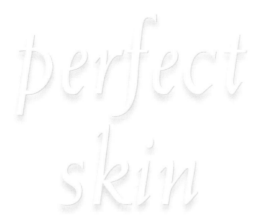

Days 17–21
5 DAYS OF ENERGISING AND REFINING

DAY 17

Clearing congestion

For the face ~ After morning or evening cleansing, massage with a stimulating massage oil like **Rosy Glow Face Oil** (see page 81) using the gentle manual lymphatic drainage techniques on page 89 to clear away any congestion.

For the body ~ Begin the day with alternate hot and cold showering followed by 5–10 minutes of body brushing. Using gentle, smoothing strokes massage your arms, legs, tummy and back (where you can reach) with stimulating body oil such as **Warm-up Body Oil** (see page 83) working in the direction of lymph flow. Repeat the massage again in the evening after a warm bath or shower.

DAY 18

Toning up

For the face ~ As for day 13.

For the body ~ In the morning use hot and cold showering followed by body brushing. Gently massage a body-refining gel or lotion such as

Lemon Refining Lotion (see page 91) into the skin.

In the evening take a warm bath or shower but finish with a quick cold blast. Pat dry then massage gently in the direction of lymph flow with **Warm-up Body Oil** (see page 83).

DAY 19

Re-defining

For the face ~ As for day 13.

For the body ~ In the morning use hot and cold showering, followed by body brushing. Gently massage **Lemon Refining Lotion** (see page 91) into the skin. In the evening, stimulate lymphatic drainage with the Feet Treat on page 89.

DAY 20

Zone control

For the face ~ After cleansing, apply **Rosy Glow Face Oil** (see page 81) but begin to incorporate stimulating massage movements such as scissoring and brisk circling movements into your routine to stimulate blood flow.

For the body ~ In the morning use hot and cold showering, followed by body brushing and then apply **Lemon Refining Lotion** (see page 91).

In the evening take a warm bath or shower, then spray the breasts and bottom with cold water for a few minutes. Pat dry and rub **Lemon Refining Lotion** or a specific bust-firming preparation like **Uplifting Gel** (see page 93) into the breasts. Massage cellulite-prone hips and thighs with an anti-cellulite oil such as **Contour Smoothing Massage Oil** (see page 93). Use deep, stroking movements in the direction of lymph flow.

DAY 21

Energising

For the face ~ As for day 16.

For the body ~ In the morning use hot and cold showering, followed by body brushing and then apply **Lemon Refining Lotion** (see page 91).

In the early evening take an energising bath.

Add infusions of stimulating herbs like lavender, rosemary, peppermint and thyme to the bathwater or use **Instant Energy Bath Oil** (see page 83). Finish by spraying all over with cold water and then apply **Uplifting Gel** (see page 93) to the breasts and massage cellulite-prone areas with **Contour Smoothing Massage Oil** (see page 93). You can now begin to use more stimulating massage movements like kneading, squeezing and percussion (see page 81).

Energising supplements

- Take ginseng tonic 3 times a day, or every other day, if you begin to feel over-energised and agitated. Do not drink coffee at the same time as taking ginseng.

- Drink 25ml (5 teaspoons) wheatgrass or watercress juice.

- Treat yourself to a couple of professional manual lymphatic drainage treatments.

- Try a Thai massage.

Days 17–21: *daily revitalising plan*

- Soon after waking, drink a cup of hot water and the juice of a freshly squeezed lemon.

- Begin the day with a full-body stretch. Stand with the legs apart and arms loosely by your side. Slowly raise your arms above your head and stretch up, lifting on to your tiptoes. Hold for at least 10 seconds, then drop your arms. Now bend from the waist downwards so your head and arms hang loosely down and reach towards your toes.

- Breathe deeply – follow the exercise on page 79 each day. Choose a time when you are unlikely to be disturbed.

- Season your meals with plenty of stimulating and lymph-cleansing foods such as ginger, cinnamon, garlic and parsley.

- Drink at least 1 litre (1³/₄ pints) of fluids (mostly pure spring water) a day, including 3 cups of ginger juice. To prepare this, make 425ml (³/₄ pint) of pressed pineapple juice up to 570ml (1 pint) with pure spring water and pour into a saucepan. Add a good chunk of fresh ginger root (2.5cm/1in square) and warm gently for about 10 minutes.

  Alternatively, add about 30g (1oz) of sliced fresh ginger to 570ml (1 pint) of water, bring to the boil and simmer for 15 minutes. Then add a good squeeze of fresh lemon juice and sweeten with honey.

- Aim to do 20–30 minutes of aerobic exercise a day. This can be anything from brisk walking to jogging.

- Before bedtime, stretch. Lie on your front with your hands flat on the floor by your sides at chest level. Push up with your arms, open your chest and stretch your head back to look at the sky. Hold for at least 10 seconds. Tuck your head in and slowly roll back so you are sitting on your knees but with your arms stretched out in front of you and forehead to the ground – as if in prayer. Hold for 10 seconds then come out of the stretch slowly.

Days 22–28
7-DAY SKIN-PERFECTING PROGRAMME

Daily skincare extras

Day 22 ~ Exfoliation for face; sea salt bath.

Day 23 ~ Moisture boost (see Day 5 or 7); massage cellulite-prone areas.

Day 24 ~ Steam treatment – for face and body.

Day 25 ~ Hydrotherapy bath with herbs or essential oils to soothe or invigorate depending on how you feel.

Day 26 ~ Scalp or foot massage to aid relaxation.

Day 27 ~ **Seaweed Bath** or **Seaweed Body Wrap** (see page 46).

Day 28 ~ Nourishing skin treatment – apply **Nourishing Serum** (see page 70) or a face mask.

Daily maintenance from within

- Drink 1 litre (1³/₄ pints) of pure spring water a day, beginning and ending the day with a glass.

- Sprinkle four-seed mix on to breakfast cereal or over yoghurt to get your full complement of skin-moisturising essential fatty acids.

- Eat at least 1 large salad a day including vegetables in all the rainbow colours.

- Take at last 30 minutes of exercise (preferably outdoors) a day.

- Enjoy a glass of freshly squeezed fruit or vegetable juice every day.

- Add in anything from this programme that has proved particularly beneficial to you.

> ### Daily skincare essentials
>
> Morning stretch.
> Morning cleansing ritual.
> Hot and cold showering.
> Body brushing followed by
> **Lemon Refining Lotion**
> (page 91).
> 20-minute mini meditation
> or dream visualisation.
> Evening cleansing ritual.
> 5-minute face massage.

attune

CHAPTER ELEVEN

Troubleshooting

~

The Essence of Problem-free Skin

Skin problems are upsetting. When skin is marred by blackheads and spots or dry scaly patches, perfection is always just out of reach. Yet these upsets are often a tell-tale sign that something is out of kilter. Every problem has a story to tell and we can learn to interpret these messages. A holistic approach considers all the contributing factors and aims to bring skin back into balance. The secret of keeping skin healthy and happy is to heed and respond to its distress signals.

Be attuned.

BLACKHEADS AND CLOGGED PORES

Dark, enlarged pores are a sign of congestion. They appear when sebum, the skin's natural oil, becomes lodged in the thin duct leading from the glands to the pores. Sebum is actually a

---
— Recipe —
CLEAR SKIN SCRUB

1 tablespoon hazelnut oil
1 teaspoon jojoba oil
1 tablespoon finely ground almonds
5 drops lemon, juniper or patchouli essential oil

Mix the hazelnut and jojaba oil in a small glass bowl. Add in the almonds and stir well. Finally, drop in the essential oil.

Massage this scrub into your skin concentrating on the sides of the nose, chin and between the eyebrows or wherever the blackheads are clustered. Leave on the skin for 5 minutes. It may also help to melt the congested sebum by gently steaming the face by filling a bowl with just-boiled water, bending over it and covering your head with a towel. Sponge clean with warm water and wipe away oily residues with cottonwool soaked in witch hazel or orange flower water.

---

liquid wax and when trapped it begins to solidify.

Oily skin tends to be more susceptible to blackheads because the sebaceous glands are especially active. However, congestion only arises when the free flow of sebum is stifled. The blockage is usually caused by sticky dead cells lining the duct or by superficial flaky cells that are not being sloughed away properly. The dark colour is often regarded as dirtiness but is actually due to melanin pigment within these cells.

As sebum's job is to form a watertight film on the skin, blackheads often go hand-in-hand with dryness. Over-washing is not the answer. It won't shift congested sebum and makes the skin even drier.

Holistic solutions

- Adding oil to an oily skin may sound like madness. However oil dissolves in oil, not water. The way to clear the congestion is to slough away any flaky cells blocking the pores and melt away the sebum. Try the scrub on the left.

- Essential oils such as lavender, lemon, lime, orange and geranium help to regulate the activity of the sebaceous glands. Add 1–2 drops of your favourite essence to a teaspoon of aloe vera gel and apply to problem areas every morning and evening.

🌢 At least once a week use a deep-cleansing mask like **Peppermint Purifying Mask** (see page 27) to help draw out deep-seated impurities.

🌢 Eat lots of beta-carotene-rich foods such as carrots, apricots, cantaloupe melon, pumpkin and spinach. This nutrient is converted into vitamin A, which is known to normalise the way cells are shed. It can help to shift blockages and helps to prevent pores from becoming congested.

🌢 Congested skin often reflects congestion within. If you are frequently constipated, bulk up your diet with lots of wholegrain cereals, fruits and vegetables. For fast relief try infusing a teaspoon of psyllium seeds or linseeds in a cup of boiling water and sip when cool.

SPOTS AND PIMPLES

Even perfect skins fall victim to the occasional spot or pimple. However, spots invariably spring from blocked pores. When sebum accumulates in the duct (hair follicle), bacteria which normally live quite harmlessly in the sebaceous ducts start to multiply. The bacteria produce toxic chemicals that provoke inflammation so the whole area becomes red and feels tender.

The body then sends white 'infection-fighting' blood cells into the ducts or hair follicles to kill the bacteria. As the fight ensues, pus forms and the follicle becomes even more inflamed. Eventually the pus bursts on to the surface, carrying cellular debris with it.

When inflammation occurs deep within the follicle, pus cannot escape resulting in a sore lump that takes several days to go down. The reason squeezing is taboo is because it can force the infection inwards, creating just this sort of problem. Deep-down inflammation also carries a risk of scarring.

Spots have a habit of appearing when least wanted, for instance before a special event like a wedding day or party. Stress may have some-thing to do with this. Excess adrenaline often nudges the sebaceous glands into hyper-drive. Inner tensions also interfere with the processes of elimination and toxins may end up being pushed out through the skin. Spots are more likely to occur in the pre-menstrual phase, sug-gesting a hormonal link-up.

People who keep their anger bottled up inside often suffer from spots. This emotion upsets the liver, the organ responsible for clearing toxins from the blood, which may help to explain why.

Holistic solutions

- Follow the guidelines for reducing blackheads, to help keep spots at bay.

- Cleanse your skin with a foaming wash or milky cleanser containing tea tree and lavender essential oils. These essential oils have antiseptic and anti-bacterial properties which help to keep the spot-forming bacteria in check.

- If you feel a spot forming, dab a drop of pure lavender essential oil on to the tender area. This is the only essential oil that can be used undiluted. Do this several times a day.

- As spots often indicate the need for inner detoxing, drink a glass of hot water and the freshly squeezed juice of half a lemon as soon as you get up each morning for a week. This will help to cleanse and tone the liver.

- If spots appear when you are feeling run down, it could be a sign that your immune system is in need of a boost. As well as being an effective immune tonic, the herb echinacea is also renowned for helping to clear up spots. Try taking 15–20 drops of echincea tincture in glass of water three times a day for ten days.

- If you are apprehensive about a future event, be sure to meditate or do a visualisation each day. It may just help to keep any spots at bay.

ACNE

Most people experience the odd spot once in a while, but acne is a very different affair. This is a complex inflammatory condition which seems to be triggered by a hyper-sensitivity to androgen hormones, namely the male hormone testosterone.

Acne is most common during puberty when hormone levels are in flux. However, this sudden sensitivity can be sparked off at any time of life. The over-responsive sebaceous glands then react to androgens by going into overdrive and causing an oil crisis. This sets the scene for blackheads and spots to form. Experts suggest the propensity to get spots occurs because the cells lining the follicles are particularly sticky and when they die they clump together creating a blockage, as opposed to flowing away with the oil. Others suggest changes in the consistency of sebum may contribute to this state of congestion. There is also a special breed of bacteria responsible for creating spots known as *Propionibacterium acnes*. In mild cases the skin may have a splattering of blackheads and just a few spots. When acne is more severe, the skin is hyper-sensitive, inflamed and the spots are so infected that they turn into pustules and cysts.

Why the skin suddenly becomes so sensitive remains a mystery but stress, especially the competitive variety, may play a role. High-flying career women were among the first to develop acne in later life. Acne also flares up in times of stress.

Holistic solutions

As acne is characterised by sensitivity, treatment should focus on calming and soothing as well as gently clearing away excess oil and keeping skin bacteria under control.

- Avoid harsh cleansing routines. Opt for a gentle, non-perfumed foaming wash, vegetable soap or cleansing milk to clear away dirt and other debris.

- Don't use abrasive skin scrubs. Wipe skin with a little freshly squeezed pineapple juice diluted with pure spring water to dissolve away congested cells.

- Gently massage the skin with an oil containing essential oils like neroli, lavender, myrrh, juniper, thyme, camomile and patchouli (see **Acne Soothing Oil**, right). Remove residues with a tissue soaked in witch hazel or orange flower water.

- Keep acne bacteria in check with tea tree essential oil. Add 1–2 drops to a teaspoon of aloe vera gel and apply lightly all over the problem areas. You can also dab individual spots with some neat lavender essential oil.

- Hot, humid conditions tend to make acne worse so avoid steaming and Turkish baths. The dry heat of a sauna may be helpful, but if acne is aggravated by heat give it a miss. Treating skin to regular clay-based masks can help to draw out ingrained impurities.

- Acne often improves in sunlight. Waves of red and blue light activate chemicals called porphyrins which kill bacteria. UV rays are also mildly anti-bacterial and in small doses have immune-boosting properties.

- Encourage inner cleanliness with plenty of freshly squeezed juices. Try combinations of

---

– Recipe –
ACNE SOOTHING OIL

2 teaspoons hazelnut oil
1 teaspoon calendula oil
1 teaspoon jojoba oil
2 drops neroli essential oil
1 drop camomile essential oil
1 drop myrrh essential oil

Blend all the ingredients together in a small glass bowl, then decant into a tinted glass bottle. Massage on to the skin at least every other day, preferably daily. Tissue-off excess and tone with witch hazel. Keeps fresh for up to 6 months.

carrot and watercress, apple and mango, apricot and cherry, plus the occasional shot of wheatgrass for a purifying boost.

§ Certain nutrients are often low in acne sufferers. These are vitamin A (or beta-carotene), vitamin E and zinc. Ensure your diet supplies plenty of these important skin foods. As raspberries, strawberries, cherries, blackcurrants, redcurrants and black grapes contain anti-inflammatory flavonoids, they may also prove helpful.

§ Avoid foods rich in hard, saturated fats and be sure to get enough liquid essential fatty acids. They may influence the quality of your sebum.

§ Find time to unwind. Bouts of stress trigger acne flare-ups so, for your skin's sake aim to feel calm and composed. Flower remedies may offer emotional support. Crab Apple (Bach Flower) is very good when you feel unclean and full of self-loathing.

BROKEN CAPILLARIES AND THREAD VEINS

Fair, delicate skins are particularly vulnerable to broken capillaries and thread veins which resemble tiny red squiggles beneath the surface. Although the minute capillaries that feed skin are buried in the dermis, they become visible when the epidermal layer is thin and translucent. Broken veins on the cheeks and nose give skin a ruddy appearance. Often these tiny capillaries are not broken, but their walls are fragile so they dilate and blood collects inside them. Sometimes they do actually rupture and minute quantities of blood seeps into the tissues.

Exposing fragile skin to harsh environmental conditions such as intense cold and heat is not a good idea. High blood pressure and some drug medicines, such as steroid and hydrocortisone creams which cause skin to become thinner, may exacerbate the problem.

Holistic solutions

§ Cleanse the skin with preparations containing soothing herbs such as camomile. Try making your own **Camomile Scented Milk** (see page 21) and refreshers from infusions of camomile or marigold flowers.

§ Choose a rich moisturiser that will form a protective barrier between your skin and the elements. Again opt for those containing infusions of camomile and marigold flowers.

§ Essential oils with strengthening qualities, such as rose, cypress and camomile, are good for broken capillaries so add a few drops to your moisturiser. Massage

166

vulnerable areas with special treatment oil made by adding 6 drops of your chosen essential oil to 1 tablespoon of calendula oil.

❧ Bioflavonoid compounds present in plant foods help to strengthen capillaries and, being potent antioxidants, protect the fragile walls from free-radical damage. Find them in the pith of citrus fruits such as lemon, orange and grapefruit, green peppers, beetroot, papaya and berry fruits such as cherries, black grapes, blueberries, strawberries and blackcurrants. Aim to drink a glass of freshly squeezed whole orange or grapefruit juice each day.

❧ Avoid anything that makes the capillaries dilate, such as hot, spicy foods, alcohol, coffee and cola drinks. Rosehip and camomile teas are good substitutes.

❧ Add lots of fresh parsley to salads and cooked dishes. It is an excellent source of vitamin C and bioflavonoids needed for good capillary health.

❧ Never subject fragile skin to temperature extremes. Avoid plunging it in hot water, having steam treatments or spraying it with hot and cold water.

CHAPPED OR ROUGH SKIN

There are times when skin can lose so much moisture that it becomes rough and cracked. Dehydrated skin not only feels very uncomfortable, but is also susceptible to infections. Chapping happens when skin's protective barrier has broken down and can no longer prevent moisture escaping to the atmosphere. Areas of skin with very few sebaceous glands are particularly vulnerable. The lips, for example, have none.

But this is just part of the story. Skin only becomes this dehydrated when its barrier is also eroded by eternal factors such as over-washing in harsh alkaline detergents and/or exposure to harsh environmental elements like bitter winds and parching sun.

As our hands are washed several times a day and are out in all weathers, they can easily become chapped during the winter months.

Holistic solutions

Nip dryness in the bud by bolstering skin's natural barrier with a rich and protective moisturiser – the creamier the better. Be sure to apply your lip balm or handcream frequently, i.e. before venturing outside and immediately after washing your hands. See recipe for **Minty Lips**, page 39.

For an intensive softening hand treatment prepare an infusion of comfrey or marshmallow root and soak both hands in this warm solution for ten minutes or more. Pat dry with a tissue and then massage or preferably soak them in a little warmed olive or avocado oil for a further ten minutes.

Tissue off the excess oil then apply lots of **Sandalwood Softener** (see below). For best results, put on a pair of cotton gloves overnight or for a few hours in the day so the cream really has a chance to soak into the skin.

Dry skin indicates a need for more essential omega 3 and 6 fatty acids. During the winter months try to add 3 tablespoons of cold-pressed and uncooked vegetable oils such as flax, hemp, pumpkin seed, walnut or soya oil to your diet. Use them to make salad dressings and vegetable dips, and drizzle over steamed vegetables and baked fish in place of melted butter.

– Recipe –
SANDALWOOD SOFTENER

1 teaspoon white beeswax
1 teaspoon cocoa butter
1 teaspoon emulsifying wax
2 tablespoons avocado oil
2 tablespoons marshmallow root infusion
6 drops sandalwood essential oil

Melt the beeswax, cocoa butter and emulsifying wax in a small bowl over a saucepan of simmering water. When liquified, stir in the avocado oil with a wooden spoon and when well blended stir in the marshmallow root infusion. Remove from the heat and allow to cool, stirring occasionally. Finally stir in the sandalwood essential oil and decant into a glass jar. Keeps fresh for up to 4 weeks when chilled.

CELLULITE

Like everything, cellulite is easier to prevent than treat (see page 95). For most of the year, cellulite is out of sight and also out of mind. Only when summer looms do we panic and set about banishing these lumps and bumps with a short-lived orgy of pummelling and punishing dietary regimes. Needless to say most of these efforts are doomed to failure.

Cellulite is notoriously stubborn and by the time skin takes on that orange-peel appearance without needing to be squeezed, it is not going to disappear overnight. But don't despair. There is lots you can do that will make a difference, providing you persevere.

Holistic solutions

As a variety of different factors contribute to the build-up of cellulite, the best way to tackle this problem is to address them one by one. Be prepared – it will take between four to six weeks to see a real difference in smoothness and tone.

- Oestrogen encourages fat and fluids to be deposited in the hip and thigh area, so taking steps to restore hormone balance is a priority. Phyto-oestrogens may be helpful as they lessen the impact of excess oestrogen. Good food sources are legumes such as soya, chickpeas, mung beans and lentils.

- The liver is responsible for neutralising and clearing toxins from the body. After winter it is always rather sluggish. Start the day with the juice of half a freshly squeezed lemon in hot water. Sip three cups of specially formulated detox tea during the day (for stockists see page 199). Eat liver-cleansing foods such as artichokes, ginger, garlic, dandelion leaves and grapefruit.

- Cellulite begins when the blood flow to the fat cells falters, so aim to improve circulation in stricken areas. Strengthen the capillaries by eating plenty of antioxidant-rich fruits and veg-etables, especially berry fruits. Sip black grape juice or take *Vitis vinifera* (extract of grapes and vineleaves). Both are rich in flavonoids and tannins that improve capillary health.

- Poor lymph drainage means fluid stagnates in cellulite-stricken areas. If you are really serious about shifting these lumps and bumps, treat yourself to a course of four to six manual lymphatic drainage treatments.

- Drink lots of water and prepare meals with fluid-flushing vegetables and herbs such as celery, dandelion leaves, fennel, tarragon and parsley.

- Once a week take a **Seaweed Bath** and smother problem areas with a **Seaweed Body Wrap** (see page 46). Add stimulating essential oils of rosemary, lavender and lemon to potentise seaweed and ordinary baths. Body brush the skin after baths and

— Muscle toning —

Toning the muscles of the bottom and the inner and upper thighs will help to redefine this area when used in combination with aerobic-style exercise.

1. Lie on your side with legs stretched out, your head resting on the lower arm and the upper arm resting on the floor. Lift the upper leg 15cm (6in), hold for 10 counts, then gently lower. Repeat this 20 times, then roll over on to the other side and repeat the exercise.

2. Kneel on all fours with your back straight. Lift one leg up behind you, keeping it bent, and feel the bottom muscles working. Do this 20 times then repeat with the other leg.

– Recipe –

ANTI-CELLULITE GEL

2 tablespoons aloe vera gel

2 tablespoons green tea

20 drops bladderwrack tincture

20 drops ivy tincture

6 drops rosemary essential oil

6 drops lemon essential oil

6 drops juniper essential oil

Spoon the aloe vera gel into a bowl, stir in the green tea and finally drop in the tinctures and oils. Keeps fresh for 1 week when chilled.

then massage **Anti-cellulite Gel** (see above) into problem areas.

🌢 What you eat and drink definitely makes a difference. Stick to your healthy eating blueprint and avoid salty and sugary foods. Sugar and refined carbohydrates are easily turned into fat which is stashed away on the hips and thighs. Sprinkle seaweed into salads, soups and stir-fries to give your metabolism a boost, eat plenty of fresh vegetables and fruits, stay away from alcohol, coffee and strong tea. To help shift those stubborn fat cells drink green tea instead.

ECZEMA

Characterised by extremely dry, inflamed and itchy skin, eczema is a very common problem that affects one in ten of us. When eczema develops early in life, it is mainly referred to as atopic and usually runs in families with a history of allergies such as hayfever and asthma

Certain household allergens such as dust, house-mites and animal danders seem to provoke flare-ups. Outbreaks of eczema can also be triggered by viral infections and stress. Eczema usually appears on the inner arms, especially elbows, backs of knees and wrists but in severe cases may affect the whole body. Sometimes tiny itchy blisters appear and the skin can be weepy. Scratching itchy eczema can allow germs to pass into the skin which leads to infection.

Eczema also occurs when the skin reacts to certain irritants such as nickel in jewellery, perfumes and plastics. This may also be referred to as contact dermatitis. Hydro-cortisone cream and steroid drugs bring relief by switching off the allergic response and giving skin a chance to heal, but as soon as treatment ceases the problem recurs. Long-term use of hydro-cortisone creams makes the skin thinner and more easily damaged. It is impossible to remove inherited tendencies but there is lots you can do to prevent flare-ups and keep eczema at bay.

170

Holistic solutions

- Cleanse skin with the mildest soapwort cleanser. If cracked and weepy, avoid using essential oils as they may act as irritants. Try applying a compress, made by soaking muslin in an infusion of camomile, to itchy and inflamed areas.

- Put a good handful of oatmeal into a muslin bag and hang from the bath tap so softening extracts seep into the water.

- If the skin flares up, massage with a soothing and strengthening blend of nourishing oils morning and evening, see right.

- Eczema-prone areas need intense moisturising. First apply some pure aloe vera gel to the skin, then overlay with a rich moisturiser. The balm recipe (right) contains ingredients that are valuable for treating eczema.

- The omega 3 and 6 fatty acids are particularly helpful for eczema sufferers. As well as moisturising skin from within, they also reduce inflammation. It is well worth supplementing your diet with a combination of cod liver oil and borage oil capsules. Zinc, vitamin C and B6 are also important nutrients for promoting skin healing.

- As stress aggravates eczema, finding a way to stay calm and composed helps keep flare-

— *Recipes* —

ECZEMA SOOTHING MASSAGE OIL

30ml (2 tablespoons) apricot kernel oil
1 teaspoon calendula oil
10 drops borage oil
10 drops wheatgerm oil
6 drops sandalwood or patchouli essential oil

Mix the oils together in a small glass bowl, then add the essential oil. Keeps fresh for up to 6 months.

ECZEMA SOOTHING SKIN BALM

1 teaspoon white beeswax
1 teaspoon cocoa butter
1 teaspoon emulsifying wax
1 tablespoon apricot kernel oil
1 teaspoon calendula oil
1 teaspoon borage oil
2 tablespoons pure spring water
6 drops sandalwood or patchouli essential oil

Melt the beeswax, cocoa butter and emulsifying wax in a glass bowl over a saucepan of boiling water. Slowly pour in the calendula and borage oils with a wooden spoon and then add the water. Remove the bowl from the heat and allow to cool, stirring occasionally. Finally add your essential oil. Store in a tinted glass jar. Keeps fresh for up to 4 weeks.

ups at bay. Be sure your diet is rich in anti-stress B vitamins.

- Chinese herbal medicine is often successful at treating skin problems such as eczema. Treatment is specially tailored to each individual and eczema has been known to clear completely.

- Reduce exposure to dust and house-mites as well as any known allergens. Investing in anti-dust-mite bedding often reduces eczema flare-ups. Wear pure cotton, silk and soft natural fibres next to your skin – avoid prickly wool. Food allergies can also trigger and exacerbate eczema.

PSORIASIS

This skin condition seems to be genetic and whilst it can be cleared and kept under control, like eczema it has a propensity to flare up from time to time.

Psoriasis is characterised by raised circular patches of pink and flaky skin. These occur because cell turnover goes haywire. For some unknown reason new cells are produced at around ten times the normal rate and as they stack up, they give rise to these rough patches of skin. The condition is made worse by stress as well as cold, damp conditions. However, when

steps are taken to improve overall health, for example inner cleansing, nourishing and relaxation, psoriasis frequently clears.

Holistic solutions

- Cleanse skin gently with a simple infusion of soapwort. Coal tar is renowned for regulating cell turnover and the soap may be helpful when used in moderation.

- Include infusions of herbs such as comfrey, camomile and marshmallow in your moisturising cream. Herbalists also swear by the external use of white willow bark and inner bark of elm for treating psoriasis. Tie these herbs up in muslin and soak in the bath.

- The Dead Sea cure is renowned for its ability to clear up psoriasis. Numerous different elements appear to work in combination. These include bathing in the sulphur rich springs at Ein, being immersed in the Dead Sea, having body packs of Dead Sea mud and soaking up the sun's rays (at this low-lying location there is very little burning UVB and a much higher proportion of UVA).

  At home Dead Sea salts can be added to baths and Dead Sea mud can be used as a body treatment.

- Avoid getting over-stressed. The relaxing

atmosphere at the Dead Sea has its part to play in this healing cure.

- Although sunbathing is generally ill advised, psoriasis does seem to improve with exposure to strong sunlight. It is worth remembering that sun damage catches up in later life so be cautious and never allow your skin to burn.

- Eat plenty of foods rich in beta-carotene which is converted into vitamin A, a nutrient involved in the smooth transition of new skin cells to the surface. Along with vitamin E it helps to regulate cell renewal and prevent flakiness.

- Consider taking supplements of cod liver oil (rich in vitamin A and essential fatty acids) or an oil rich in omega 3 and 6 fatty acids such as linseed (flax) oil. Nibble on walnuts and pumpkin and sunflower seeds.

- Some psoriasis sufferers find their skin improves when they avoid coffee, citrus fruits, corn, milk and tomatoes. Prescribed drugs, including anti-malarials and painkillers, may also provoke flare-ups.

- Try sipping cups of Redbush or Rooibos tea and adding a pot of infusion to bath water. This popular South African folk remedy is rich in flavonoids with anti-inflammatory and anti-allergic properties.

EYES (PUFFINESS)

Under-eye puffiness occurs when fluid collects in the tissues just beneath the eyes. Like dark shadows under the eyes, a tendency towards puffiness is often inherited. Other contributing factors are poor lymphatic drainage and sluggish kidneys. Both problems are worse for lack of sleep, drinking too much alcohol and stress. As the skin becomes thinner and less elastic with age and sun damage, puffiness appears more pronounced so wear a good pair of protective shades in strong sunlight.

Holistic solutions

- Avoid using heavy rich preparations which may drag on the skin. Gels are ideal for the day (see **Rose and Aloe Eye Gel** page 38), but as skin ages a lightweight moisturising cream like **Rose Petal Moisturiser** (page 38) may be better for the night

- To help the fluid drain away, try lying with your head supported by a neck roll instead of a pillow at night and avoid sleeping in centrally heated rooms without opening a window.

- Gently tapping with the fingertips, working from the nose outwards, helps to dispel puffiness and is more effective when coupled with plant-rich eye preparations.

🌢 Applying eye masks can help to tone and refine skin in this area. Slices of raw potato are a tried and tested folk remedy for relieving slight puffiness. An attractive alternative are cottonwool pads soaked in rose water.

🌢 Both puffiness and under-eye shadows can be minimised by helping the kidneys. Avoid coffee and strong tea. Instead drink plenty of pure spring water, sip herbal infusions from purifying herbs such as burdock and ursa uvi, add kidney-toning plants such as fennel, dandelion leaves and watercress to salads.

SCARS AND STRETCH MARKS

Skin has amazing regenerative powers. If skin is damaged by cuts, burns or tears the epidermal cells and dermal fibres can knit back together again. However, in doing so scar tissue forms which has a slightly different colour and texture. These scars do fade with time but their imprint may last a lifetime. With sore, acne-type pustules inflammation is often deep-seated and, if infection is pushed deeper into the skin by squeezing, skin may be permanently scarred by such spots.

Stretch marks are essentially deeper-lying scars. When skin is over-stretched, collagen fibres in the dermis may rupture. This is most likely to happen during pregnancy or when weight is rapidly gained and lost. Newly forming collagen and elastin fibres repair the damage but leave silvery lines behind. Typically stretch marks appear on the hips, stomach, bottom and upper thighs.

Holistic solutions

🌢 If your body shape is changing through diet, exercise or pregnancy be sure to keep the skin supple and well lubricated (see **Supple Skin Oil** on page 122). Other essential oils that are good for reducing stretch marks are neroli and mandarin.

🌢 When René Gattefosse (the father of modern aromatherapy) burnt his hand in a lab experiment, he instinctively plunged it into a nearby vat of lavender oil and was amazed at how rapidly his skin healed without scarring.

Lavender is known for its healing properties, but many other essential oils including rose, camomile, neroli and geranium help wounds to mend faster and minimise scarring. The sooner skin is treated, the better. Lavender is the only essential oil that can safely be applied neat

– *Recipe* –
SKIN REPAIRING OIL

1 tablespoon sweet almond oil
1 teaspoon calendula oil
1 capsule vitamin E oil
2 drops lavender essential oil
2 drops geranium essential oil
1 drop myrrh essential oil

Blend the ingredients together and massage into damaged skin twice a day for 4 weeks, then once daily until the skin is well healed. Keeps fresh for up to 6 months.

to cuts and burns. Old scar tissue has been known to improve with regular applications of essential oils. Try the recipe above.

- Vitamins C and B6, zinc and sulphur are closely involved in the healing process and ample supplies help skin repair itself more effectively. Preparations containing these nutrients may also promote skin healing when applied externally. Creams containing methyl sulphonyl methane (naturally occurring sulphur) are being successfully used in the treatment of burns, scars and acne, while creams enriched with soluble vitamin C have a soothing effect on traumatised tissue, reducing inflammation and speeding healing.

SENSITIVE SKIN

In Britain around 80 per cent of women say their skin is sensitive or easily provoked to redness and irritation. The usual advice is to opt for hypoallergenic preparations which contain fewer potential allergens.

Sensitivity, however, is not the same as a true allergy. An allergic response is provoked by a specific trigger such as pollen with hayfever. It can be any natural or synthetic substance including herbs and essential oils. When the allergen is inhaled or comes into contact with the skin, the cells pour forth the arch-irritant histamine. This gives rise to swelling, inflammation and itching which causes skin to erupt in weals characteristic of nettle rash or urticaria. Allergic reactions are intense but short-lived and symptoms usually subside in a few hours. Re-exposure to the allergen sets the whole process in motion again.

In contrast, sensitive skin reacts in a non-specific way to a variety of substances that are well tolerated by normal skins. Sensitive skins become vulnerable because their natural defences have been gradually eroded.

Close examination reveals that the stratum corneum is excessively porous. It allows water to pass out, making skin feel taut, and irritants to move in. Sensitivity also suggests the body is trying to cope with too many toxins. These may come from your diet, from medication and from environmental chemicals. From the skin's point of view over-treatment with a variety of different skincare preparations each containing 20 or more chemical ingredients may be too much for it to handle.

– Recipe –
SOOTHING SKIN BALM

1 teaspoon white beeswax
1 teaspoon cocoa butter
1 teaspoon emulsifying wax
1 teaspoon avocado oil
1 teaspoon grapeseed oil
1 teaspoon calendula oil
10 drops evening primrose oil
2 tablespoons camomile or comfrey infusion
1 tablespoon aloe vera gel
6 drops camomile or sandalwood essential oil

Melt the beeswax, cocoa butter and emulsifying wax in a bowl over a saucepan of simmering water. Slowly stir in the oils with a wooden spoon. When blended, stir in the herbal infusion. Remove from the heat and allow to cool, stirring occasionally. When the mixture is lukewarm, blend in the aloe vera gel and add the essential oil of your choice. Keeps fresh for up to 4 weeks when chilled.

A holistic approach to treating sensitivity lies in streamlining your skincare regime, using pure and simple preparations, bolstering skin's natural defences and detoxing from within.

Holistic solutions

§ Use a gentle and simple cleanser such as **Scented Milk** made with rose or camomile (see page 21), then spray with rose water or an infusion of camomile. Never use a toner containing alcohol on sensitive skin.

§ Moisturise with a cream that soothes and rebuilds the skin's natural defences. Try the **Soothing Skin Balm**, left. Dab a little of each ingredient on your skin first to check if it is an irritant.

§ Treat your skin from within by following a gentle detox programme. Stay away from coffee, alcohol and cigarette smoke.

§ Boost your intake of omega 3 and 6 essential fatty acids to strengthen your skin's natural barrier from within (see page 54).

§ Choose organically grown foods rich in antioxidant nutrients such as vitamin C, beta-carotene, vitamin E and zinc which help to boost your protection from within. Black grapes, blueberries and cherries are rich in flavonoids, phytonutrients with antioxidant and anti-inflammatory properties.

SUNBURN

Providing you know how sun sensitive your skin is, take steps to bolster its natural defences and avoid excessive exposure, burning should not occur. However, it may be difficult to gauge the burning power of the sun. If in doubt always overprotect because sunburn is to be avoided at all costs.

When skin receives an overdose of UV radiation, free radicals are generated which rampage through the epidermal cells. They respond by releasing chemicals which cause inflammation and swelling. Burning is not immediately obvious. It may be four to six hours before the skin starts to turn pink. It then becomes progressively more hot, prickly and can be agonising.

If a large area of skin is burnt, water is lost through the skin and this can lead to dehydration, even heat-stroke. In some cases blisters appear and although the burning sensation subsides in two or three days, the skin may then start peeling to get rid of damaged cells.

Badly scalded areas of skin are sites where skin cancers often develop, albeit many years later. There is evidence that sharp sunburn shocks, especially in childhood, increase the risk of developing skin cancer so it is essential to protect children's fair skin.

If you do get sunburnt, stay out of the sun until the pinkness and pain have disappeared. If you do venture out, cover up sunburnt areas completely and, even after the sunburn has faded, slather these areas with a high SPF sunscreen.

Prevention is the best solution, see page 136.

Holistic solutions

- Be sure to use enough sunscreen – you will need at least 1 teaspoon for your face to get adequate coverage. Applying too thinly reduces the actual SPF. Remember to reapply at least every hour.

- Help take the heat out of the skin with tepid baths and showers.

- A folk cure for sunburn involves applying natural yoghurt to the skin. Aloe vera gel also soothes inflammation and replaces lost moisture. Add 6 drops of healing lavender essence to a tablespoon of aloe vera gel and dab a little on to burnt areas.

- Drink lots of pure spring water and freshly squeezed juices to replenish lost fluids and minerals.

- Flood the skin with antioxidants from within and without. Try bathing burnt areas with green tea or make a compress by soaking muslin in the tea, wringing out the excess and laying over the skin. Creams containing vitamin C may help to undo some of the damage caused by burning.

essentials

CHAPTER TWELVE

Skincare Essentials

~

Our skin has a special affinity with all things natural. Elements sourced from land and sea have amazing powers for unleashing its natural beauty. Discover the purifying properties of clays and muds from the ocean depths, the cleansing qualities of milk, the gentle healing power of honey and the skin-quenching benefits of aloe vera. Learn about the nourishing oils, therapeutic herbs and sweet-smelling essential oils that bring out the best in your skin. Knowing nature's secrets is the key to formulating your perfect skincare regime. Let your imagination run wild.

Be inspired.

Beauty Comes Naturally

Why attempt to make your own skincare preparations when there are so many good-quality cosmetic creations to choose from? Here are six good reasons.

The real thing ~ It's a bit like comparing a home-cooked meal using the best and freshest natural ingredients and ready-prepared 'convenience' food. When making skincare preparations at home you use only the finest quality natural ingredients. These are fresh and free from preservatives, colourings and artificial fragrances which might irritate your skin.

Assurance of purity ~ If you want skincare preparations that are guaranteed organic (that is free from any trace of chemical pesticides), the best way is to make them yourself using organically certified vegetable oils, herbs, essential oils, honey and milk.

Best for you ~ By choosing the ingredients that go into your cleansers, moisturisers and masks, you can tailor preparations to suit your own skin and its individual needs. Play around with the ingredients as the seasons change to ensure your skincare regime delivers just the right degree of cleansing and protection for you.

Simplicity ~ Home-made cleansers, creams and masks are made with just a handful of ingredients compared to those made commercially. As a result, they are less likely to provoke sensitivity reactions. Doing it yourself means you know exactly what goes into your preparations and you can test each ingredient individually to be sure it doesn't upset your skin.

Inexpensive ~ Natural ingredients are for the most part very reasonably priced. The most expensive items are essential oils but, being highly concentrated, a small bottle will last for months. The recipes make small quantities which ensures your preparations are always fresh and there is little wastage.

It's fun ~ Making your own skincare creations is quick, easy and, like cooking, enormously satisfying. Home-made products can be just as effective as those that come neatly boxed and packaged for your convenience.

Still not convinced? Try it out and see for yourself.

Essential Basics

The following are the pure, natural ingredients needed to make superb
cleansers, moisturisers, masks and bodycare preparations.

Once you have these basics to hand you are one step closer to perfect skin. For information on stockists, see pages 197–9.

Aloe vera

From the rubbery leaves of this desert cactus plant comes a juice with exceptional moisturising and healing properties. Native Americans traditionally used poultices of aloe vera to reduce inflammation and soothe sunburn. Aloe vera juice is rich in antioxidant vitamins, essential amino acids and minerals such as calcium, magnesium, manganese, zinc, potassium and copper.

Other phytonutrients include saponins with mild antiseptic properties and anthraquinones which are anti-viral, antibiotic and anti-inflammatory, plus a hormone that accelerates wound healing.

As a gel, aloe vera is a helpful treatment for many skin conditions such as eczema, acne, psoriasis, hives, boils, burns and cuts.

Beeswax

A hard white or cream-coloured wax made by honey bees. An essential ingredient in moisturisers and nourishing creams, this wax acts as a thickener and emulsifier. It contains a mixture of fatty acids and esters that combine with oils to form an effective watertight film on the skin's surface. I've specified white beeswax in the recipes because I prefer white-coloured cream but either is fine to use.

Cocoa butter

The beans from the cocoa or chocolate nut tree yield a rich, buttery substance that has wonderful skin-conditioning and softening qualities. Cocoa butter brings a quality of richness to creamy cleansers and moisturisers. It comes as buttery coloured flakes or in solid chunks rich in palmitic and oleic fatty acids.

Emulsifying wax or ointment

A white waxy substance that enables oil and water (including herb and flower infusions) to blend. Essential when making milks and creams. Without emulsifying wax the ingredients will curdle and congeal.

Fuller's earth

A soft brown clay with amazing powers of absorption, it is highly valued for its deep-cleansing properties. When used in face and body packs it draws out deeply ingrained impurities. Fuller's earth is particularly rich in silica and other minerals which may to some extent be taken up by the skin. Useful as an occasional deep cleanse for normal and oily skins; not recommended for fragile or delicate complexions.

Glycerine

A sweet, transparent, honey-textured liquid with humectant or water-attracting qualities. Added to creams it increases their moisturising power and prevents them from drying out. Glycerine can be made from animal or plant material, so if you want to create animal-friendly preparations be sure to choose vegetable glycerine.

Green clay

Clays were used by Egyptians, Greeks and Romans to detoxify the system, heal wounds, relieve athletic aches and pains, rejuvenate the skin and promote a sense of wellbeing. Green clay is one of the most useful cosmetic clays with its purifying, toning and revitalising properties. Containing a wealth of minerals and trace elements such as silica, magnesium, titanium, iron and calcium, it coaxes oily and dry skins towards normality. Green clay's healing and slightly antiseptic properties make it good for clearing congestion and blemishes. An ideal base for home-made masks.

Honey

Made by bees from nectar and other plant substances, honey is 98 per cent sugars (fructose and glucose) and 2 per cent enzymes, vitamins and minerals. Honey has long been prized for its skin-softening and moisturising qualities. One of honey's constituents, inhibine, has mild antiseptic properties making it helpful for treating acne-prone skin.

The best varieties are cold-pressed as heating destroys essential enzymes. Slight cloudiness indicates a high concentration of vitamin-enriched pollen. Honey brings harmonising, healing and calming qualities to face masks and creams.

Kaolin

One of the finest clays, kaolin is a white powder with mild astringent qualities. As well as lifting impurities from the skin, it also improves lymphatic flow and increases blood circulation to the area. It is purifying and revitalising and best for normal to oily skins. Kaolin combines well with yoghurt, honey and fruit in face masks.

Milk

Cleopatra, the celebrated Egyptian queen, knew the beautifying properties of milk. This natural emulsion of oil droplets suspended in a watery solution (whey) makes milk a wonderful natural cleanser. As well as clarifying, milk nourishes and moisturises to leave skin silky soft. Research shows that the proteins in milk also stimulate the production of new collagen in the dermis to keep skin looking and feeling younger. For skin treatments choose whole milk as essential oils dissolve in the oily globules – try to use organic milk. Milk smells so much nicer when scented with rose or jasmine. If you are allergic or intolerant to cow's milk, choose goat's or ewe's milk instead. Being rich in phyto-oestrogens, soya milk may be a good choice for more mature skins.

Moor

While clays are composed of minerals, moor is essentially organic for it is made from plants broken down over many years to form a dark brown paste. One of the most famous moors comes from the Neydharting Valley in Austria. Believed to be around 20,000 years old, it is formed from over 300 different medical plants including eye-bright, golden rod, basil, mint, winter-berry, dandelion and valerian native to this area. The healing agents in these plants are reputedly preserved in the moor. Applied to the skin, moor cleanses, neutralises bacteria, reduces inflammation and speeds healing. Added to baths, moor appears to increase circulation, oxygenation and may even help to restore hormone balance.

Mud

Muds are primarily used in spas as deep-heat treatments. They are mixed to a paste and applied warm to the skin so as to boost the blood flow and induce perspiration. Good for revitalising dull and sallow-looking skin.

Enriching mud with nourishing vegetable oils and essential oils can enhance its therapeutic powers. Smooth over areas in need of revitalisation, leave for 5–10 minutes before rinsing off. Avoid areas with broken capillaries or veins.

The rich black mud harvested from the bed of the Dead Sea has unique qualities which reflect its unusual origins. The Dead Sea is technically a land-locked lake located at 394 metres below sea-level at the deepest geological depression on the earth's surface. This arid area is bathed in intense sunlight which promotes excessive evaporation so the sea salts are ten times more concentrated than those present in ordinary seawater. The mineral composition is also different with a higher proportion of potassium, magnesium and bromide ions, which appear to have a soothing and sedating influence on the nervous system. This may explain why the Dead Sea mud and salts can benefit skin conditions like psoriasis, acne and eczema which are aggravated by stress. For home treatment, Dead Sea salts can be added to the bath while the mud can be used as a skin treatment.

Yoghurt

When milk is spiked with bacteria such as *Lactobaccilus acidophilus* and *Bifidobacteria bifidum*, it turns to yoghurt. Eating 'live' yoghurt favours the presence of friendly bacteria in the gut which in turn promote healthy digestion. When applied to the skin, lactic acid (made from lactose sugar by the bacteria) acts as a mild exfoliator for sloughing away dead skin cells. Yoghurt brings clarifying and moisturising qualities to face masks. Also apply neat to the skin to soothe sunburn.

ESSENTIAL HERBS

Let these therapeutic plants coax your skin back into balance. The herbs I've chosen are renowned for their skin-perfecting qualities. You can use these herbs as simple cleansers or toners, incorporate them into skin creams, add them to face and body masks, or soak them in your bath. Many can also be taken as tisanes and tinctures to evoke beauty from within.

Camomile (*Matricaria chamomilla*)

This herb has small daisy-like flowers that smell like newly mown hay. Contains azulene, a soothing, anti-inflammatory chemical that promotes healing. Soothes irritable skin conditions such as eczema. Benefits combination and sensitive skins. See also Essential Aromatherapy Oils, page 191.

Comfrey (*Symphytum officinale*)

This is also known in country lore as knit-bone. Rich in soothing and healing allantoin, comfrey encourages cuts and bruises to heal without scarring. Helpful for acne and smoothing wrinkles. Benefits oily, normal and combination skins.

Echinacea (*Echinacea angustifolia*)

A statuesque plant with purple daisy-like flowers. Sipped as a tea it cleanses blood and lymph as well as supporting the immune system. Helps to clear spots and blemishes through inner cleansing. When applied externally, echinacea speeds tissue repair. Benefits spots, acne, slow-healing wounds and mild burns.

Elderflower (*Sambucus nigra*)

This plant has subtly perfumed, creamy white flowers. Elderflower water is an old remedy for refining skin, removing freckles and keeping skin blemish-free. Helpful in a steam facial for clearing blackheads. Benefits sallow skin and wrinkles.

Horsetail (*Equisetum arvense*)

One of the richest plant sources of silica, a nutrient that keeps skin soft and supple. Helps to firm and strengthen skin when used externally. Helps prevent stretch marks and smooth away cellulite. Benefits oily skin and skin problems such as acne and eczema.

Jasmine flowers (*Jasminum officinalis*)

A heavenly perfumed, natural aphrodisiac. Jasmine infusion is a good floral refresher. Benefits dry and sensitive skins. See also Essential Aromatherapy Oils, page 192.

Lady's mantle (*Alchemilla mollis*)

A valuable herb for women. Sipped as a tea it is helpful for menstrual disorders such as period pains. On the skin it soothes chapped, sore and itchy skin. Benefits dry, sensitive skin and wrinkles.

Lavender (*Lavandula officinalis*)

This plant has misty violet flowers with a cool distinctive aroma. Sipped as a tea it has a calming and rebalancing influence on the nervous system. Good for skin problems exacerbated by stress. Promotes healing. Benefits oily, sallow and blemish-prone skins. See also Essential Aromatherapy Oils, page 192.

Lemon balm (*Melissa officinalis*)

A fragrant herb with a lemony smell, uplifting yet calming. As a tea it is a useful tonic for the heart, circulatory and nervous systems. Relieves tension. On the skin it helps reduce redness and soothe inflammation. Ideal for normal and sensitive skins.

Lime blossom (*Tilia europaea*)

Also known as linden, this herb has gentle tranquillising qualities when sipped as a tea. On the skin it promotes healing and smoothes wrinkles. Helpful for eczema. Benefits normal and ageing skins.

Marigold (*Calendula officinalis*)

A plant with brilliant orange flowers and amazing powers to soothe and heal. It encourages burns, cuts and blemishes to heal without scarring. Mildly antiseptic. Benefits oily skins.

Marshmallow (*Althaea officinalis*)

A soothing and healing herb with moisturising properties. Helpful for treating eczema, boils and slow-healing wounds. Smoothes wrinkles. Ideal for dry, sensitive skin.

Meadowsweet (*Filipendula ulmaria*)

A sweet-smelling herb rich in iron and calcium that helps to preserve a sense of balance. Ideal for combination and dry skins.

Peppermint (*Mentha piperita*)

This herb has a distinctively refreshing, clean and uplifting aroma. A stimulating herb with decongestant properties. Good for clearing blackheads. Makes a cooling skin refresher for the summer months. Ideal for normal and oily skins. See also Essential Aromatherapy Oils, page 193.

Rose (*Rosaceae*)

A soft, feminine aroma. The petals have cooling and soothing properties. Infusions are helpful for itchy, inflamed or sunburned skin. Rosehips (berries of the wild rose) are one of the richest natural sources of vitamin C. Rosehip oil will help heal scar tissue. Ideal for virtually all skin types. See also Essential Aromatherapy Oils, page 193.

Rosemary (*Rosemarinus officinalis*)

This plant has small purple flowers and an intensely refreshing and stimulating aroma. Revitalises and helps boost the circulation. Helpful for shifting cellulite. Ideal for sallow and oily skin preparations. See also Essential Aromatherapy Oils, page 193.

Sage (*Salvia officinalis*)

A plant with soft, silvery coloured leaves with a distinctive aroma. As a tea, sage promotes and normalises menstrual cycles. Helps relieve excess perspiration and is also recommended for menopausal hot flushes. Unsafe to take during pregnancy. Relieves puffiness linked to pre-menstrual tension. May help shift cellulite and helps treat eczema.

Soapwort (*Saponaria officinalis*)

The root, resembling fine wood chippings, gives rise to a decoction (see opposite) that is one of the gentlest natural cleansers. A true soapless

– Preparing herbs –

- Infusions/tisanes – use 1 tablespoon of dried herb in approximately 570ml (I pint) of water or 1 heaped teaspoon to a cup of water. Place the herb in a cup or small basin and pour boiling water over it. If making a tisane, leave to steep for 5–10 minutes before straining and drinking. For skin preparations leave to stand for at least one hour or until cool. Strain through a coffee filter before using in skincare preparations. For fresh herbs use double the quantity.

- Decoctions – for tougher parts of the plant such as roots, berries, bark and seeds. Use the same quantities as for infusions but add a little more water to allow for loss through evaporation. Place the herb in a ceramic or enamel saucepan, pour water over and bring to the boil. Simmer for 3–5 minutes, remove from the heat and strain before drinking. For skincare preparations allow to steep for at least one hour before straining.

- Tinctures – are alcoholic solutions containing the active principles of herbs and plants. Tinctures tend to be stronger than infusions or decoctions. The usual dose is 10–20 drops taken in a wineglass of water. Tinctures can also be added to skincare preparations in place of infusions and decoctions.

soap. Adding aromatherapy oils can tailor this lotion to suit your skin type. Ideal for dry, sensitive skins and acne.

St John's wort (*Hypericum perforatum*)

Recently acclaimed as a natural antidepressant, this plant bearing bright golden flowers has long been prized for its skin-enhancing qualities. On the skin, hypericum soothes swelling and encourages healing of cuts, burns and wounds. Helpful for sunburn and rashes. It may cause photosensitivity so don't apply before going out in the sun. See also Super Supplements, pages 189–90.

Yarrow (*Achillea millefolium*)

One of the oldest healing plants, yarrow was used as a first-aid treatment by warriors. As a tea it promotes circulation and has diuretic properties, but should be avoided during pregnancy. Infusions of yarrow cleanse and help to heal wounds. Helpful for treating acne and skin blemishes. Ideal for oily and problem skins.

ESSENTIAL NOURISHING OILS

Pure plant oils work wonders at nourishing, softening, lubricating and protecting the skin. They are essential ingredients of cleansing milks and creams, moisturisers, face masks and as carriers for aromatherapy or essential oils.

Apricot kernel oil

Pale yellow oil with rich, nourishing properties. Contains vitamins (A, B1, B2, B6 and E) and minerals (calcium, phosphorus, potassium and sulphur). Helps calm inflammation and irritation. Helps treat eczema and dermatitis. Benefits all skins especially dry and sensitive types.

Avocado oil

Dark green, often slightly cloudy oil from the cold-pressed flesh of avocados. Rich in vitamins, antioxidants and minerals. Cools and calms inflammation. Helps treat eczema. Benefits all skins, especially dehydrated and mature types.

Grapeseed oil

Pale green-yellow colour, very pure and with an exceptionally light, fluid texture that quickly sinks into the skin. Grapeseed extract is a potent antioxidant. Rich in omega 6 linoleic acid and vitamin E. Benefits normal and oily skin types.

Hazelnut oil

Golden yellow oil containing a good spectrum of vitamins and minerals. Slightly astringent qualities and penetrates quickly. Helps treat acne. Benefits normal, oily and blemish-prone skins.

Olive oil

The health and beauty benefits of this rich green oil have been harnessed for centuries. Rich in vitamin E and other phytonutrients preserved only in the cold-pressed virgin varieties. Soothes and calms inflammation. Helps heal burns and scars. Best when blended 50:50 with a lighter oil like grapeseed. Benefits all skin types especially those that are dry and devitalised.

Sweet almond oil

Very pale yellow oil rich in vitamins, minerals and protein. Softening and nourishing. Soothes parched and chapped, itchy and inflamed skin. Helps treat eczema and other skin irritations. Benefits normal and dry skins.

Soya oil

Pale-coloured oil extracted from soya beans. This is one of the few good sources of essential omega 3 (alpha-linolenic) as well as omega 6 (linoleic) fatty acids, both needed to form cell membranes responsible for keeping moisture in the skin. Soya oil is light-textured and easily absorbed. Helps treat acne. Benefits all skins, especially oily types.

Sunflower oil

Exceptionally light, pale golden oil with little aroma. In addition to vitamins and minerals, it is one of the richest natural sources of omega 6 linoleic acid. Easily absorbed into the skin. Benefits all skin types.

SUPER SUPPLEMENTS

These are oils with special therapeutic properties that benefit a variety of skin conditions. They are rich and should be used sparingly (10 per cent dilution in other nourishing oils).

Borage oil

Also known as starflower oil, this golden oil comes from the seeds of borage flowers. One of the richest known sources of gamma-linolenic acid (GLA) which is exceptionally good for the skin. (The body makes GLA from omega 6 linoleic acid but conversion may be hindered by dietary deficiencies, alcohol and ageing.) Helps treat symptoms of pre-menstrual tension as well

as psoriasis, eczema and prematurely aged skin. Regenerating. Benefits dry, ageing skin.

Calendula oil

Made by steeping marigold flowers (calendula) in organic sunflower oil. Creates a richly coloured oil with cooling and healing qualities. Rich in carotene and saponins. Soothes inflammatory conditions such as eczema. Helps reduce scarring. Benefits damaged and aggravated skin.

Carrot oil

A bright orange oil, extracted from carrots, with cleansing and healing qualities. Rich in the orange pigment beta-carotene. Helps clear spots and blemishes. Offers mild protection from sunburn and helps develop a tan when mixed with sesame oil. Helps prevent dryness, burns and repairs sun-damaged skin. Benefits ageing skin and wrinkles.

Evening primrose oil

Extracted from the seeds of the evening primrose flower, a favourite herbal remedy amongst Native Americans. A good source of GLA. Helps dry skin conditions and helps rebalance sebaceous secretions, so well worth including in a daily moisturiser. Keeps skin looking youthful. Benefits psoriasis and eczema.

Hemp seed oil

A green oil that comes from the seeds of the marijuana plant. Boasts a perfect balance of the two essential fatty acids (omega 3 alpha-linolenic and omega 6 linoleic, as well as useful quantities of GLA). A relative newcomer provoking interest for its beneficial effects on dehydrated, prematurely aged skin and eczema.

Hypericum oil

St John's wort flowers are steeped in olive oil, then exposed to sunlight for three weeks to create a rich, deep red oil with soothing, anti-inflammatory properties. Helps treat damaged skin, eczema and dermatitis. Benefits oily and angry skins.

Jojoba oil

The beans of this evergreen South American desert plant yield an oil once prized by the Aztecs who used it to protect their skin from dehydration and sunburn. Jojoba oil is technically a liquid wax that closely resembles the skin's own sebum. It is naturally anti-bacterial and helps treat psoriasis, eczema and acne. Benefits all skin types.

Macadamia nut oil

A richly textured oil from a plant native to Australia. Like jojoba, the oil has a chemical composition similar to that of sebum. Benefits dry and ageing skin.

Sesame oil

A slightly greasy texture, but absorbs UV radiation and offers the best sun protection of all vegetable oils. Rich source of omega 6 linoleic acid as well as various vitamins, minerals, lecithin and amino acids. Helps treat skin disorders such as eczema. Benefits all skins in the sun.

Wheatgerm oil

A rich, golden viscous oil that is an exceptionally rich source of vitamin E, a potent antioxidant that protects essential fatty acids from oxidation. Good to include in skincare preparations as a preservative. Helps treat eczema, psoriasis and prematurely aged skin. Benefits dry skin and wrinkles.

Essential Aromatherapy Oils

These oils embody the aroma of scented plants and have many
therapeutic and skin-beautifying qualities.

Essential oils are very concentrated – it takes around 200kg (440lb) of fresh flowers to make just 1kg (2·2lb) of oil – so use them sparingly to lend your skincare preparations a pleasant aroma as well as boosting their potency. They should never be used neat on the skin – always blend with a carrier oil.

Choose and use the oils whose scent you find attractive – there is no pleasure in wearing a cream that smells repellent to you – as well as considering which is best for your skin. Aim to have about ten favourite oils in your basic repertoire and gradually build up.

Basil

A tonic for the nervous system with antiseptic properties. Good for relieving stress-induced fatigue and anxiety. Helps to normalise menstrual cycles. Use in revitalising baths or massage oils for skin that develops spots before a period.

Camomile

A soothing and calming essence. Good for problems related to nervousness, over-excitabil-

ity and irritability. Helps allergic conditions and pre-menstrual tension and irregular periods. Benefits sensitive skin and conditions such as acne, rashes and eczema.

Frankincense

Also known as olbanum, the use of this rich, resinous essence dates back into antiquity. The ancient Egyptians certainly knew of its skin regenerative and anti-ageing powers. One of the most healing oils, it is also slightly sedative and antiseptic. Soothes inflammation and redness. A wonderful aid to meditation. Benefits ageing skin and wrinkles.

Geranium

A sweet-scented energy tonic for restoring natural vitality. Helpful for menstrual problems and fluid retention. Stimulates circulation, soothes itching and promotes healing. It also has rebalancing qualities and helps repel biting insects. Good for treating all kinds of skin problems such as acne, burns, cuts, bruises and eczema. Benefits all skin types.

Ginger

A warm and spicy essence with stimulating and aphrodisiac qualities. Helps to boost the circulation, especially during the colder months. Benefits cellulite-prone skin.

Jasmine

A heavenly perfume that combines beautifully with ylang ylang, neroli and rose. Soothing and energising. Renowned as an aphrodisiac, jasmine lifts the spirits. It also encourages tissue repair, calms inflammation and eases pain. Try massaging it into the tummy to reduce labour pains. Benefits oily, mixed and sensitive skins.

Juniper

A pungent and detoxifying essence. Promotes healing, soothes inflammation and keeps bacteria in check. Diuretic and circulation-stimulating properties make it good for preventing and treating cellulite. Helps to treat stretch marks and skin problems like psoriasis, eczema and acne. Benefits oily and blemished skin.

Lavender

A cool and fragrant essence with remarkable powers to heal. Calms and revitalises. Boosts the circulation. Encourages skin repair, reduces inflammation and relieves irritability. Helps to treat burns, cuts, acne, eczema and swelling. Good for keeping cellulite at bay. Benefits all skin, especially oily types.

Lemon

A fresh, citrusy aroma with uplifting and stimulating qualities. Astringent, antiseptic and rejuvenating properties make it helpful for treating congested skins prone to blocked pores, blackheads and spots as well as wrinkles. Stimulates circulation and is good for broken capillaries and thread veins. Benefits oily and ageing skin.

Myrrh

Like frankincense, myrrh has been used for centuries. It is a superb healer with anti-inflammatory properties. Helpful for treating very chapped, cracked skin and eczema. Regenerative and possessing hormone-like properties make it good for keeping wrinkles at bay. Benefits dry and ageing skins.

Neroli

Extracted from the fragrant blossoms of the bitter orange tree, this essence not only smells divine but is incredibly therapeutic too. Tranquillising and peace-instilling qualities make it good for stress-induced skin problems. It also encourages a good night's sleep, so add to evening baths and include it in preparations used before bedtime. Good for broken capillaries and poor circulation as well as preventing stretch marks and wrinkles. Normalises sebaceous secretions making it good for oily and dry skin. Benefits all skin types, particularly ageing and problem skins.

Nutmeg

A warming, spicy and reviving essence useful during the winter months. Stimulates circulation and is good to include in invigorating body oils. Combines well with orange. Helpful for keeping cellulite and general fatigue at bay.

Orange

This comes from the same bitter orange tree as neroli but is extracted from the citrus fruits. Rejuvenating essence that is good for reducing wrinkles, especially those due to the sun. Helps to treat acne and eczema. Benefits sallow and ageing skin.

Palmarosa

A cooling essence with lemony overtones. Gentle yet antiseptic, it is useful for treating acne and will help to clear scars left behind by spots. Good for broken capillaries. Benefits dry, ageing and problem skins.

Patchouli

A musky smelling essence widely used in India with healing and anti-bacterial properties. Soothes inflammation. Helpful for treating acne, eczema and dry, cracked skin. Benefits problem skins.

Peppermint

A cool and refreshing essence containing menthol. Reduces swelling and stimulates the circulation which helps keep cellulite at bay. Cleansing and antiseptic qualities make it good for skins prone to spots. May be too irritating for sensitive skins. Benefits oily and sallow skins.

Rose

A quintessentially feminine essence with skin-perfecting qualities. Calms, cools and reduces inflammation. Good for normalising periods and lifting the spirits. Helps relieve puffiness, especially around the eyes. Soothes sensitivity and clears tiny broken capillaries. Benefits normal, dry and delicate skin.

Rosemary

A truly aromatic essence with stimulating qualities. Good for banishing tiredness in both mind and body. Boosts circulation and is a useful ingredient in energising body oils. Helps keep cellulite at bay. Benefits dull, lifeless skin.

Sandalwood

Has been used as a perfume and medicine in India for centuries and remains one of the main Ayurvedic remedies. A gentle, soothing oil with moisturising and antiseptic qualities. Helpful for treating damaged, chapped skin and acne. A wonderful aid to meditation. Benefits all skins, especially dry, sensitive types.

Tea tree

This oil comes from the leaves of a tree native to Australia and boasts potent antiseptic, anti-viral, anti-fungal and anti-bacterial qualities. Seems to act selectively to disarm pathogenic bacteria while leaving the friendly skin bacteria unharmed. Helpful for treating and preventing spots, fungal infections, burns and acne. Benefits skin prone to blemishes.

Ylang ylang

Prized for its delightful perfume, this oil also has soothing and relaxing qualities. Good for all kinds of stress-linked skin conditions. Wearing preparations made with this essence help you to keep your cool. Benefits most skin types.

IMPORTANT NOTE

Just because these ingredients are natural and largely therapeutic does not guarantee that they will not cause irritation or allergy. Any substance may upset your skin so it is best to test a little on a patch of skin before adding it to your skincare preparations.

Buying Cosmetics

If you still feel, for whatever reason, that you don't have time to make your own cosmetics, then look for products with similar ingredients to the recipes.

Always check labels carefully. Certain substances and chemicals used in making cosmetics are known to be irritant and don't appear to do your skin any favours.

Cosmetic ingredients to avoid

Mineral oil (petrolateum) ~ A cheap, low-grade petroleum oil devoid of any nutritional value although widely used in moisturisers and anti-ageing creams. May provoke adverse reactions to sunlight and strips away the skin's own natural oils leading to dry skin and chapping. Encourages premature ageing.

Mono, di and triethanolamine ~ Used as thickeners and to adjust pH in facial cleansers. These chemicals appear to possess hormone-disrupting properties. They irritate eyes, provoke allergic reactions and cause skin dryness.

Parabens (methyl, propyl, butyl and ethyl) ~ Preservatives that prolong shelf-life and inhibit microbial growth. Toxic substances that cause many allergic reactions and skin rashes.

Propylene glycol ~ Often made from synthetic petrochemicals or from mixing vegetable glycerine with alcohol. Used as a humectant to moisturise the skin. A key ingredient in anti-freeze. Can cause allergic and toxic reactions.

Sodium lauryl sulphate ~ A synthetic degreaser used in foaming washes. Can cause eye irritations, skin rashes and allergic reactions.

Synthetic colours ~ Added to disguise or enhance the shade of the final product. They are labelled as FD&C or D&C followed by a colour number. Potentially cancer-causing and should be avoided at all costs.

Synthetic perfumes ~ 99 per cent of the 5,000 chemicals in perfumes are made from petrochemicals. They include benzene derivatives and air-polluting aldehydes. Petrochemicals penetrate the skin and accumulate in the fatty tissue where they may cause toxic reactions such as headaches, dizziness, rashes and skin irritations.

Reading List

Atlas of the Human Anatomy, Marshall Cavendish, 1985

Boyle, Mike, Indge, Bill and Senior, Kathryn, *Human Biology*, Collins Educational, 1999

Chu, Dr Anthony C and Lovell, Anne, *The Good Skin Doctor*, HarperCollins, 1999

Cochrane, Amanda and Harvey, Clare, *The Encyclopedia of Flower Remedies*, Thorsons, 1993

Davies, Dr Stephen and Stewart, Dr Alan, *Nutritional Medicine*, Pan Books, 1987

Fairley, Josephine and Stacey, Sarah, *The Beauty Bible*, Kyle Cathie, 1997

Gittleman, Ann Louise, *Before the Change*, Harper San Francisco, 1998

Hepper, Camilla, *Herbal Cosmetics*, Thorsons, 1987

Kenton, Lesley, *The New Joy of Beauty*, Vermilion, 1995

Lee, John R, *Natural Progesterone*, Jon Carpenter Publishing, 1996

Little, Kitty, *Kitty Little's Book of Herbal Beauty*, Penguin, 1980

Lowe, Professor Nicholas and Sellar, Polly, *Skin Secrets*, Collins & Brown, 1999

Marks, Professor Ronald, *Psoriasis*, Martin Dunitz, 1981

Marks, Professor Ronald, *The Sun and Your Skin*, Optima, 1988

Marsden, Kathryn, *Superskin*, Thorsons, 1996

McKie, Professor Rona, *Eczema and Dermatitis*, Martin Dunitz, 1983

Neal's Yard Remedies, *Make Your Own Cosmetics*, Aurum Press, 1997

Orton, Christine, *Eczema Relief*, Thorsons, 1986

Roddon, Louise, *Skin Deep*, Headline, 1995

Ryman, Danièle, *The Encyclopedia of Plants and Oils and How They Help You*, Piatkus, 1991

Sharon, Dr Michael, *Nutrients A-Z*, Prion Books, 1998

Wheater, Caroline, *Juicing for Health*, Thorsons, 1993

Worwood, Valerie Ann, *The Fragrant Pharmacy*, Macmillan, 1990

Stockist Information

Absolute Aromas Ltd
2 Grove Park
Mill Lane
Alton
Hampshire GU34 2QG
Tel: 01420 540400
Fax: 01420 540401
e-mail: oils@absolute-aromas.com
Good range of essential oils, vegetable oils, oil burners, bottles and jars.

Aromantic
22 Drumine Road
Forres
Morayshire IV36 3YY
Tel: 01309 692000
e-mail:
aromatics@bigfoot.com
Natural skincare preparations, oils and clays

Aveda
Tel: 020 7410 1600 for information on stockists
website: www.aveda.com for location of your nearest Aveda Lifstyle Store or Salon.
Eco-conscious skincare products made from pure plant and flower ingredients – free from petrochemical derivatives.

Baldwins
173 Walworth Road
London SE1 1RW
Tel: 020 7703 5550
website: www.baldwins.co.uk
Pure vegetable soaps, organic essential oils and loose herbs, herbal tinctures, flower remedies, carrier oils, floral waters, skincare essentials such as beeswax, emulsifying wax and cocoa butter, jars and bottles.

Bioforce Ltd
Olympic Business Park
Dundonald
Ayrshire KA2 9BE
Tel: 01563 851177
e-mail:
enquiries@bioforce.co.uk
website: www.bioforce.co.uk
Top-quality herbal tinctures cultivated and made in Switzerland.

The Craven Clinic
54 Cambridge Grove
Hammersmith
London W6 0LA
Tel: 020 8563 8133
e-mail:
kcampion@globalnet.co.uk
Superb detox tea with 16 different herbs created to an old yogic recipe, *herbal tonics for blood cleansing, liver, kidneys, etc. Natural-bristle brushes and superfood supplements.*

Cariad Ltd
Rivernook Farm
Sunnyside
Walton on Thames
Surrey KT12 2ET
Tel: 01932 269921 (mail order)
e-mail: sales@cariad.co.uk
website: www.cariad.co.uk
Essential oils, vegetable oils, blends for bath and body, creams and lotions, pure vegetable soaps scented with essential oils, flower waters and Dead Sea salts.

Findhorn Flower Essences
Mercury
Findhorn Bay
Forres
Morayshire IV36 0TY
Tel: 01309 690129
e-mail:
info@findhornessences.com
website:
www.findhornessences.com

Flower Essence Repertoire
The Working Tree
Liphook
Hampshire GU30 7JS
Tel: 01428 741572
e-mail: flowers@atlas.co.uk
website: www.ifer.co.uk
Offers an extensive range of flower remedies and essences from across the world including Australian Living Flower, Flower Essence Society, Australian Bush, Master's Flower Essences, Deva Flower Elixirs and Findhorn Flower Essences.

Healing Herbs
P.O. Box 65
Hereford HR2 0UW
Tel: 01873 890218
e-mail: healingherbs@healing-herbs.co.uk
website:
www.healing-herbs.co.uk
Bach flower remedies made in the traditional way.

Higher Nature
Freepost Licence No T.N. 7289
Burwash Common
East Sussex TN19 7BR
Tel: 01435 882880 (orders)
Fax: 01435 883720
e-mail:
sales@higher-nature.co.uk
High-quality supplements, oils (flax) and aloe vera.

Jurlique
Willowtree Marine
West Quay Drive
Yeading
Middlesex UB4 9TA
Tel: 020 8842 3956
e-mail: Info@Jurlique.co.uk
website: www.jurlique.co.au
Natural skincare products created by Dr Jurgen and Ulrike Klein made primarily from herbs and flowers home-grown organically in South Australia, along with other organic ingredients. No chemicals, artificial preservatives, colours or fragrances.

Knots Elementals
29 St James's Avenue
Hampton Hill
Middlesex TW12 1HH
Tel: 020 8941 0759 (mail order)
Fax: 020 8941 2629
e-mail: mailorder@knotselementals.com
Selected essential oils and carrier oils, tinctures, floral waters, herbal soaps, sea salt for bathing and skincare bases made from pure plant ingredients.

Martha Hill
The Old Vicarage,
Laxton
Near Corby
Northamptonshire
NN17 3AT

Tel: 01780 450259
Customer Service: 0800 980 6664
e-mail:
service@marthahill.com
website: www.marthahill.com
Comprehensive range of herbal skincare products for face and body. Made with herbs, essential oils and vegetable oils.

Natural Health Remedies
10 Bamborough Gardens
London W12 8QN
Tel: 0800 074 7744
e-mail: organic@nhr.kz
website: www.nhr.kz
Certified organic aromatherapy oils, floral waters, base oils, soaps and skincare preparations.

Neal's Yard Remedies
26–34 Ingate Place
Battersea
London SW8 3NS
Tel: 020 7498 1686
Fax: 020 7498 2505
Customer Services: 020 7627 1949
e-mail: mail@nealsyard remedies.com
Organic vegetable oils and essential oils, skincare preparations, clays, beeswax, cocoa butter, vegetable soaps and natural fibre brushes.

Nutricentre
7 Park Crescent
London W1N 3HE
Tel: 020 7436 5122
e-mail: enq@nutricentre.co.uk
website:
www.nutricentre.co.uk
Wide range of supplements, herbs and tinctures, oils, clays, flower remedies and other natural products.

P.J. Cousin Herbal and Cosmetic Supplies
The London Natural Health Clinic
170 Camden Hill Road
London W8 7AS
Tel: 020 7938 3788
e-mail:
pjc@cousin.sonnet.co.uk
Oil mixes, top-quality organic oils and herbs.

Planet Organic
42 Westbourne Grove
London W2 5SH
Tel: 020 7221 7171
Organic produce, oils, vitamins, freshly squeezed juices including wheatgrass and natural products.

Revital Health Place
3a The Colonnades
123/151 Buckingham Palace Road
London SW1W 9RZ
Tel: 020 7976 6615 or 0800 252875 order hotline
Fax: 020 7976 5529
e-mail: enquire@revital.com
website: www.revital.com
Wide range of organic foods, natural supplements, herbal remedies, natural skincare products, aloe vera and flower essences.

The School of Chinese Herbal Medicine
Midsummer Cottage Clinic
Netherwestcoate
Chipping Norton
Oxfordshire OX7 6SD
Tel: 01993 830419
Can provide a register of qualified Chinese herbal practitioners.

Tisserand Aromatherapy
P.O. Box 746
Hove
East Sussex BN3 7BA
Tel: 01273 325666
e-mail: info@tisserand.com
website: www.tisserand.com
Full range of essential oils and aromatherapy preparations.

Woodspirits UK
Unit 42
New Lydenburg Industrial Estate
New Lyndenburg Street
London SE7 8NE
Tel/fax: 020 8293 4949 (mail order)
e-mail: woodspiritsuk@ compuserve.com
website:
www.woodspiritssoaps.com
Hand-made pH balanced soaps made from entirely natural ingredients including natural pigment colourings and glycerine. Biodegradable and recycled packaging.

Xynergy Health Products
Lower Elsted
Midhurst
West Sussex GU29 9JT
Tel: 01730 813642
e-mail: orders@xynergy.co.uk
website: www.xynergy.co.uk
Purest quality spirulina, biogenic aloe vera and superfood supplements.

Index